Red Light Therapy

Everything You Need to Know About Red Light Therapy

(How to Use Red Light Therapy for Fat Loss Anti-aging Muscle Gain Fatigue, and Pain)

John Demaio

Published By **Jordan Levy**

John Demaio

Red Light Therapy: Everything You Need to Know About Red Light Therapy (How to Use Red Light Therapy for Fat Loss Anti-aging Muscle Gain Fatigue, and Pain)

ISBN   978-1-998038-40-4

Legal & Disclaimer

Table Of Content

Chapter 1: What Conditions Can Light Therapy Help With? 1

Chapter 2: The Top Benefits Of Red Light Therapy 3

Chapter 3: Red Light Therapy And Cancer 20

Chapter 4: How Does Red Light Heal? 27

Chapter 5: Is Red Light Therapy Actually Safe To Use? 43

Chapter 6: Creating Space For The Treatment 50

Chapter 7: The Body Position During The Red Light Therapy 57

Chapter 8: The Position Of The Light During Treatment 63

Chapter 9: The Duration Of The Session 67

Chapter 10: Recurrence Of Sessions By Using Red Light 74

Chapter 11: Common Mistakes People
Make When Using Red Light Therapy 78

Chapter 12: Faqs About Red Light Therapy
.... 88

Chapter 13: Strategies For Accelerating
Your Healing Through The Use Of Light
Therapy... 99

Chapter 14: Tips To Get The Most Out Of
Your Red Light Therapy 113

Chapter 15: What Is Red Light Therapy?
.... 121

Chapter 16: The Benefits Of Red Light
Therapy... 124

Chapter 17: Red Light Therapy For Skin
Quality And Happiness. 127

Chapter 18: What Is Light Therapy And
How Does It Work?. 134

Chapter 19: Treatment And Tools For Light
Therapy To Help Delay The Signs Of Aging.
.... 141

Chapter 20: Does Red Light Therapy Really Work? 147

Chapter 21: How Red Light Therapy Can Make You Look Younger?...................... 158

Chapter 22: 15 Benefits Of Red Light Therapy For Your Skin. 162

Chapter 23: How To Give Yourself A Spa-Quality Red Light Peptide Facial At Home. 168

Chapter 24: The Top 3 Acne Red Light Therapy Devices.................................... 174

Chapter 25: Types/Sources Of Red-Light Therapy.. 178

Chapter 26: Benefits Of Red-Light Therapy 180

Chapter 1: What Conditions Can Light Therapy Help With?

We hear the simple fact that lighting therapy could improve our mood and assure us that we'll be to be in a position to combat a variety of diseases and disorders and illnesses, we believe this sounds odd. It is possible that we don't believe anyone who claims that it is the case. We may also be concerned over whether it works or even if it's something invented!

It is good to know that in the last century, the red light therapy and infrared treatments are being studied in depth. Research has been conducted on a wide variety of animals, as well as on human beings, to determine what effect the treatments will have on the human body. Since a large portion of the metabolic processes in cells that humans and other animals are comparable and beneficial to wellbeing of these treatments are likely to be comparable also.

There's a myriad of diverse diseases and illnesses which can be treated with using these methods in some cases, and a few studies will reveal the more as time continues. Some of these research studies have proven successful by meta-analysis as well as research reviews. Be aware that there are research studies which are controversial and might require further investigation before we're capable of proving that this is accurate.

Chapter 2: The Top Benefits Of Red Light Therapy

We are discovering more every day There are plenty of advantages that come from this type of treatment, and it's likely to be absorbed into our body and help us feel more relaxed and enhance the health of our bodies. There are however a handful of benefits you're going to discover to top the list in the majority of people who choose to give the red light therapy or any alternative light therapy, an attempt. The benefits of red light therapy are:

Melts the Belly Fat

As per the Center for Disease Control, 26.5 percent of adult population within the United States are considered obese. People who are overweight have an increased chance of developing many different ailments which can be detrimental to their overall health, such as type 2 diabetes, cancer, heart attack, stroke. In addition, the costs for medical treatment related to the conditions that are caused by being overweight will rise until weight loss.

There's an abundance of various programs which claim to assist shed weight. But it is possible using laser therapy in red could be just what you're looking for. In the year 2015, a group of researchers from the Federal university of Sao Paulo, Brazil experimented with what might result from light therapy for 64 people. The participants were split to split into two groups. One group had exercises in addition to phototherapy. The other one was just workout without any therapy with photos. It lasted for 20 weeks. Participants would have to exercise at least three times per each week.

At the completion of a workout programme, one of the participants received treatment with light, in contrast to the other who did not. The most interesting thing was the women who received treatment with light after exercising could double the fat was lost over this interval, in comparison with exercising on their own. In addition, those who had received treatment with red light observed an increase in the skeletal muscle mass when compared with the rest of the group.

An Increase in Bone Density

Bone density, or the capability of the body to create new bones with time is vital when seeking recovery from injury. This can be crucial for those who are older people, since the bones become less strong with the passage of time. It is, however, feasible to utilize the red light to boost bone density. Actually, there are a number of studies taking an examination of this such as:

2003: A study found that LLIT has a positive impact in the healing of bone-related defects implanted using inorganic bovine bone.

The study also revealed that the results of the study, together with other studies, revealed the bone was irradiated primarily by infrared light wavelengths, resulting in a variety of variables, including bone neoformation and collagen deposition. This was especially evident when compared with bones who did not receive radiation therapy in the same moment of.

The study of 2008 found that the use of lasers can improve the results in surgery on the bone. This helped in improving the outcome of any procedure of the bone. Additionally, it aid in promoting greater comfort after surgery, as well as aiding in faster recovery.

The research shows that not only will we be able be able to reap some advantages in the bones of our bodies, by building them up with treatment with light, but it will also aid us when suffering from break or any other damage to our bones. The treatment can help following surgery by enhancing the speed of recovery as well as in easing our recuperation process.

Enhances Brain Function

Nootropics have experienced a massive rise in the popularity of these drugs over time, and there is a large number of individuals that are taking these kinds of medications to increase the efficiency of their brains regarding inspiration, creativity and even memory. The beneficial effects that can be observed through red light can be seen by numerous research studies and they can prove to be safer and more effective in comparison to the nootropics.

According to researchers at University of Texas University of Texas, it was possible to use the lasers infrared near the foreheads of healthy volunteers. An experiment was conducted and the researchers analyzed how this altered the cognitive performance of those who were treated. Patients who had received the treatment noticed improvement in their memory and response time and the improvement in their positively rated emotional state after they returned for a follow-up interval following treatment.

Research has shown that this therapy is a non-invasive method to enhance cognitive functions that are related to cognition and emotional aspects.

Increases Your Levels of Testosterone

In all of history, the character of manhood has been tied to a male hormone, which is referred to in the form of "testosterone".

When you reach thirty, the majority of men notice that their levels of testosterone are declining in the hope that they'll experience adverse changes to their physical and mental health. The lower testosterone production can result in a decreased level of sexual functioning as well as a decrease in muscle mass less energy, as well as an increase in the amount of fat within the body in order to mention a few possible issues that may be encountered.

In conjunction to the notion that there are many pollutants in the environment, stress and a poor diet that affect millions of men around the globe nowadays, it's not surprising that the lower testosterone level is now becoming an issue.

The year 2013 was the time a team of Korean researchers looked into what might transpire if infrared laser light was aimed at the region of the testicular gland in males. The male rats of 30 were divided into three groups. There was one group that was controlled, followed by two others. groups were exposed to near-infrared light or red light. The experiment lasted over a period of five days.

After the test was completed in the lab, rats that weren't treated didn't observe any increase of testosterone. The animals that received an hour of daily light therapy noticed the testosterone levels raised. The rats who received the near-infrared light observed the Serum T levels increase by an impressive amount. In addition, the patients treated with red light therapy, saw almost the exact same rise during the treatment.

If you are suffering from lower levels of testosterone as well as various other health issues associated with this, it might be beneficial to take advantage of the treatment with red light. Through this method, it's possible to raise your testosterone levels while at the same time, decreasing some of the various ailments that can be associated from this condition.

Can Help You to Eliminate Depression and Anxiety

Depression and anxiety are major concerns that millions of people around the globe are grappling with each day. It is thought that 121 million individuals around the globe suffer from depression. This is merely the amount of people legally diagnosed with depression. Furthermore, it's estimated that there are more than 40 million people who are older than 18 years old in the United States alone, who have anxiety. The two issues mentioned above are in the world, however the solutions that treat them tend to be ineffective and harmful, or be a bit numbing one's mind, and worse, could create a sick person and lead to numerous health issues.

It is the reason there is certain interest in using the use of red light therapy in order to determine whether depression and anxiety can be treated by this treatment. The first step is to take a an examination of depression before we move on.

A team comprised of scientists from Harvard University tested infrared lights on ten subjects suffering from severe depression. The researchers placed the lights across the foreheads of the subjects for a single period of about 16 minutes. After just one session of this treatment, patients saw an impressive reduction in depression as well as anxiety and the most significant reduction showed after a time of 2 weeks.

The result is that near-infrared light treatment resulted in long-lasting reduction in both anxiety and depression. This is all with one treatment. Imagine what happens if you practice this method often to treat anxiety and depression!

Relieves Pain

In a research study from 2015 by the National Institute of Health, America is a land of discomfort. It is due to the fact that nearly fifty million American adult respondents said they were experiencing any kind of discomfort over the past three months. A few of the most commonly used medications for pain that people are likely to use in the event of discomfort is Ibuprofen and Tylenol. It is interesting to note that all of these medications are associated with the risk of heart attack, cancer as well as strokes. With the exception of aspirin that can lower the risk in certain situations, NSSAIDS (Non-Steroidal anti-inflammatory drugs) can be harmful to your health.

Overall, even though you feel more relaxed when you are taking these medicines but we're doing an opportunity to harm our well-being. With the aid of the infrared light therapy, you may reduce pain without the need for medication!

Heals Arthritis

Another advantage that is associated with the use of the red light therapy method is its ability to treat arthritis. It is a debilitating ailment which a lot of people across the globe are suffering from. Between 2013 between 2013 and 2015, it's estimated that 23 percent of adult patients within the United States were diagnosed with any form of arthritis. It means that approximately 55 million Americans will benefit of a the use of light therapy in order to treat them.

A Harvard professor in the Department of Dermatology, Dr. Michael R. Hamblin released a research study in 2013 that looked at how the use of red light therapy could aid in treating arthritis of patients. In the course of inducing arthritis in rats, then using only one session of red light therapy their inflammation decreased significantly in only one day. This is a great result to those suffering with arthritis and want to relieve certain pain.

Other Benefits of Red Light Therapy

It has been a long amount of the time we have spent in this section, studying the ways in which the therapy can help to enhance the health of our patients and help them get easier. There are many possibilities to be explored which will make this type therapy worthwhile. Here we will explore some of these options now.

The first thing to consider is that this procedure will assist in revitalizing your skin. Red light therapy is likely to penetrate beneath the skin, bringing increased blood circulation to the surface as well as boost your circulation. The treatment is also expected assist in increasing the production of elastin and collagen in the skin. What this does will be a healing of damaged cells that might exist, and giving the skin the appearance younger. That means the blue light will make a wonderful treatment for getting rid of any blemishes that you might have, securing the skin, as well as repairing certain damaged cells.

The next thing to consider is relief from pain. The kind of treatment will not just enhance the appearance of the skin, but it is an excellent treatment you can count on when you're in need of relief of pain. Since this treatment can penetrate deeply into your body, it's likely allow you to heal parts of cells and also. Additionally, it will also have the benefit that it can boost the amount of endorphins produced by the body. This can to block certain transmitters that can result in suffering.

A third advantage is that treatment with red light therapy could aid in rehabilitating injuries and some pro athletes who swear by how this therapy helps them be back in the sport and heal from injuries.

The reason for this form treatment is effective in accelerating recovery is because the light therapy stimulates ATP production. The chemical can lessen swelling and inflammation of the body. It also increases white blood cells. This helps to heal any tissues that have suffered damage, irrespective of what the site of damage is within the body.

The final reason why a lot of people enjoy working in the field of the red light therapy is because it may help reduce or completely eliminate acne from the body. Red light therapy is able to penetrate the skin and trigger the hemoglobin present. It will limit the supply of blood to the sebaceous glands which result in acne. This makes it more difficult for them to accomplish the job they require. The skin cells from becoming oily, and thus causing acne. If you're suffering with acne, but no other treatment options appear to work Red light therapy might be the solution is worth considering.

You can see that there's an array of health issues which can be treated by using treatment with red light. As more and more people decide to give it a go as more research is being conducted to understand how the light therapy works, and its effects on the health of your body it is likely that it is likely that you will be able to connect this therapy with a variety of different health issues. There is a chance that among the possibilities mentioned above, the this therapy will prove aid those suffering from certain health issues.

Chapter 3: Red Light Therapy And Cancer

It's important to look into the red light therapy method and consider how it could be feasible for it to assist our beat cancer. When we read this manual and discover how red light functions in the body, as well as how it's effective in affecting cells as well as the various components of our body and organs, we'll begin to learn how it can help treat various illnesses, such as cancer. First, it is important to learn more about cancer, and the ways in which it operates. The way it works may differ from the way we're used to being told or thinking about the terrible illness.

The Epidemic of Cancer

The governments of the world inform us that 50% of the people alive today will be diagnosed with a kind of cancer at some point in their lives. The most terrifying thing part of this is that should we be diagnosed with the disease treatment options that are frequently recommended to us could cause problems as well. Reminisce about the time that somebody in your life needed radiotherapy, chemotherapy or even surgery in order to treat fight cancer. Most of the time people are left with a different appearance and feel as they were prior to.

Naturally, simply researching the effects of diverse treatments tell us, it is clear they're not good. The act of cutting someone's open, introducing an element of poison into their body or even inflicting burns with the radiation produced by a nuclear weapon will, naturally, will make their condition more ill than it was before. The experiences we have as human beings have proven this over and again. It might be time to think about alternatives to consider cancer instead of using methods which might work however, they can actually hurt the health of an individual.

According the Dr. Hardin B Jones, Professor of Medical Physics of the University of California, Berkley, "My studies have proved definitively that cancer patients who are not treated are able to live for up to four times longer than treatment patients. If a person is diagnosed with cancer and chooses not to treat it in any way, he'll have a longer life span and be more comfortable when undergoing chemotherapy or radiation surgery, unless it is required in urgent life-threatening circumstances."

We are not the majority to go to this point. We are aware that treating cancer is vital and we would like to have the ability to take action to stop it. Whether you are dealing with cancer or someone else we are caring for is suffering from cancer. It is a problem that a majority treatment options currently available in the market do not work. Some of them are effective however the adverse consequences associated with them can't endure the stress of poor health.

The Metabolic Disease of Cancer

One of the biggest lies that is out there and is taught to our by the cancer industry is that a cancer cell is a tiny terrorist which has one mission with one and only one task - to take out the victim. It is believed that cancer just going to kill us If we don't take action and take drastic action in order to eliminate it is an untruth and is the root of the issue.

There's been no research which suggests that tumors or cancerous cells will cause any harm to a person however, we do get anxious and fear every time we hear "cancer". Additionally, The Cancer Genome Atlas Project which was initiated at the end of 2005, in 2005 by The National Cancer Institute, was dismissed as a fail. It did not have one single mutation in a gene, or perhaps a mixture of mutations which was determined to be in the exact position of beginning the cancer-causing process.

This might sound alarming It is due to the fact that cancer is not viewed as a genetic illness. It's been nearly 100 years since the Dr. Otto Warburg, a Nobel Prize Winning scientist, realized that a cancerous cell is a normal cell, just like the many others that are found in our bodies, and that it were damaged mitochondria by some way.

The mitochondria are small molecules inside cells accountable for creating energy for the cell. When we're discussing what we normally consider a cancerous cell it is just seeing a specific cells that are not functioning properly metabolically or is damaged and seeking repair in order to make it better.

After the Cancer Genome Atlas Project proved the fact that cancer was not a true genetic disorder rather one of metabolic origin, James Watson, known as the father of DNA suggested that we move our attention in the research regarding cancer away from area of genetics as cancer isn't the main issue we're dealing with. Instead, it is important to shift our focus towards metabolic processes and ways we will be able to treat cancer this the best way.

Knowing fundamentals of cell metabolism and how to use the information we have gained to correct metabolic problems can help to discover ways to boost the natural healing process in the body without taking medications or harmful treatments commonly given to patients with cancer. It means that we're more prepared to fight cancer, and get results, without risking our health in the course of.

Many think that infrared light therapy is among the methods that will be introduced in the future for this. This gives you the chance to utilize something naturally derived to address the root causes of cancer, and possibly stop it from happening from the beginning. It's a concept which seems absurd to many as well as some might have difficulty moving away from conventional ways treatment for the body. It's absurd that we depend on these harmful methods to fight the cancerous process, such as chemotherapy, radiation as well as surgery, rather alternatively, methods that are healthy and natural?

Chapter 4: How Does Red Light Heal?

The time has come to look into the way this red light likely to help you by helping heal your body. Trillions of cells that comprise our bodies will be able to find tiny, intimate structures in these cells, referred to by the name of "mitochondria". They are the ones responsible for the cells' energy production and are involved in the process of "metabolism".

If a cell receives enough nutrients, and even more than the amount it needs to properly process food this process which will involve the chemical oxidation of glucose to carbon dioxide in the mitochondria. This signifies that it's in good health and performing as it's supposed to do. If the depletion of metabolism in cells starts to occur, that is the time seeing more signs of disease and tumors throughout the body.

There is a fact that nearly all the major diseases that we encounter in our bodies can be traced back to the activity of mitochondria inside our cells. Knowing which food items, along with what aspects can increase metabolism and what can hinder this process the lifesaver as it will assist you in not only stop the illnesses that are occurring inside your body and even reverse some which you already suffer from.

If you undergo the Red light therapy, your skin will be subjected to lasers at a very low intensity. It is recommended to do this several times per each week and for a set period based upon your requirements. It is possible to continue this for a long time however, most individuals choose the procedure to treat specific conditions The treatment can be for a period of one to two months, until the issue is completely resolved.

You can use the red light therapy device at home, if you wish, but there's also an abundance of experts working in clinics for cosmetics or similar locations that will be competent to perform this procedure for you too. Whatever way you choose, so you make sure the appropriate tools are used you'll notice that using red light therapy can prove to be an effective method to boost your overall health.

If you are convinced of the benefits of the red light therapy consider that the lower level of this laser can help in the process of accelerating the ability for your body to heal from many illnesses, ailments and many more. Additionally, the laser helps the body boost its production of collagen and increase blood flow and help repair tissues.

We must examine at the mechanisms that this treatment is likely to function. This method of operation is very similar to that we have seen in various laser treatments. However, the red light has use a shorter frequency. It allows us to utilize the treatment on places that may be more sensitive, such as the eyes and the skin and still remain completely safe.

If we can expose our surface to this energy that it receives, it'll release more of the chemical called ATP or adenosine Triphosphate and is believed to aid the body to build new capillaries, increase collagen production and heal parts of tissues damaged by the body.

Because of this, there are plenty of occasions when people opt to utilize treatment with red light to benefit them. This therapy can assist in the treatment of problems with arthritis, treat burns, and even smooth stretch marks. This is just one possibilities of how can be used on the treatment, and we've discussed some of them, as well as the evidence that backs them with earlier in this manual.

What's interesting to note is that the initial FDA-approved application for this type of treatment and the instrument that came with it could be used to accelerate wound healing which was taking a long time. The method by which the procedure was carried out was that the red energy would be absorbed by the skin from 8 to 10 millimeters. This allowed it to be later infiltrated further inside the body. When the procedure was properly used and properly, it was able to affect the body's immune system, metabolic processes, as well as the nerve system, just to mention just a few.

We are now at the issue of why red light therapy is distinct from various types of therapies in the market. In order to simplify the treatment is going reduce to frequencies of the red light. This procedure will release some red light which can be seen, while the lasers will be released at 60 nanometers. A few of these techniques will make use of a near-infrared spectrum that is above 700 nanometers, or less visible red light. This will be more like 590 nanometers. Additionally, there are gadgets that mix red and blue light. All depends on what kind of light you select to purchase.

If we look at what we see with conventional laser therapy, we observe that these treatments produce more light with a greater density that red laser therapy. This can cause more harm to tissues in the body. It can also result in destruction, or even more so when you're not cautious. There is no risk of a concern with the treatment with red light due to the low intensity laser emits.

The purpose of conventional Laser therapy is cause damage to the skin, as it is believed that this will aid in rejuvenation and healing of the body quicker than with no procedure. It isn't will have the energy or warmth to accomplish this. You don't need to be worried about damaging, burning or burning tissues in the body. That's why it's considered to be a better treatment method than other methods.

The procedure will operate similarly to various alternative laser therapies available and the light produced by the laser will aid in the healing of the body and restore many of the cells within the body. However, it's not likely be a risky option, as it does not carry the risks that we experience with other techniques and makes it easier to utilize.

The Metabolism is being reduced by a few Toxins from the Environment

The first thing to be aware of and comprehend in relation to cell metabolism is that all the actions we be working with will be facilitated through a particular enzyme. The enzyme that is in question is "cytochrome c oxidase". The enzyme was first discovered by Dr. Otto Warburg in 1926.

Why should we know about the specific enzyme? It is the enzyme that creates the use of oxygen by cells. It is so that it is able to interact directly with the oxygen and catalyze the final step of metabolism. This is vital in order to be sure that the metabolic process of cells can take place in an appropriate way.

In his study in the field of research, the researcher Dr. Warburg found that, in the event that we can stop the enzyme involved, we could be able to take an unintentionally healthy, and turning it into cancerous. This information has been confirmed over the years by other studies and research.

This is an important discovery which we must take more time to study. If one enzyme is removed damaged, damaged, or impaired by any means, it's going to cause harm to the person. The body will struggle to perform the metabolic process it requires, which leads to the cell going from a healthy one and healthy to one with issues and may be deemed to be cancerous. According to researchers from the University of Pennsylvania in 2015, "Defects in cytochrome c oxidase expression induce a metabolic shift to glycolysis and carcinogenesis."

This is in line with what we've been discussing for years In the event that cells are not equipped with this specific enzyme or if there's additional reason for why the enzyme isn't performing what it is supposed to do it should, there could be several issues to be addressed. Cells will face health problems including cancer of all sorts as well as other. Making sure this enzyme can function according to the way it is supposed to, as well as learning how to help the metabolism operate properly can improve the overall health of your body.

There are a handful of toxins which are likely interfere with the functioning of this enzyme. These include the following: Unsaturated Fatty Acids, radiation from X-rays EVB radiation, serotonin estrogen, aluminum phosphide carbon dioxide and cyanide chemotherapy and many other. It is possible to control some of them yourself should you wish some, like the fatty acids in what you consume, however there are some that can be a little more difficult to manage.

Let's look at how they are likely to function: If you're exposed in some method to any of these environmental pollutants mentioned above in the body, cells are likely to create a radical, which is commonly referred to as "nitric oxide". The free radical will be able to directly bind to the enzyme cytochrome C oxidase, which is so needed in our lives, and will eventually be deactivated in the future. In the meantime, as long as the Nitric oxide remains attached to the enzyme this means that the cell cannot make the metabolizing process in the way that it ought to, resulting in an abnormal cancer metabolism the process.

Methods to Increase the Metabolism of Cells by Using Light in the form of red

We must consider what the red light therapy capable of accomplish to help us. The effect we're likely to observe by using near-infrared and red light on our metabolism cells is truly unique. This has prompted a number of investigations over time. Indeed, both the lights have been proven to be able to dissociate the nitric oxygen from the enzyme called cytochrome c oxidase within cells.

If the red light is effective in removing the nitric dioxide, it will do certain things that are incredible. The cytochrome C oxidase enzyme is in a position to return working, and will be much better energized. This will boost the efficiency of the enzyme. It also speeds up the metabolic process that's present, and ensure that your cell returns to its normal state rather than becoming sick and possibly cancerous. It can also cause difficulties for your.

This is a good thing for you as it indicates you will notice an increase in the way cells can process again. The cells will be able to go back to doing what they are supposed to perform naturally, something that an environmental toxin have stopped them from doing by. If this occurs, it signifies that you're likely to experience a variety of physiological and beneficial effects that will emerge in the event that your metabolic rate is increased. The beneficial results comprise:

The reduction of the amount of free radicals that are found within the cells.

The reduction of inflammation that is present throughout the body. adverse effects on condition when decrease in inflammation.

The reduction of lactic acid, which accumulates.

Reduced levels of stress hormones that are present within the body. This is something everybody will gain from.

A higher amount of CO_2 emissions.

Increased blood flow flows through the body will help us cleanse the body more easily and feel more energetic, and improve our overall general health.

A rise in the quantity of oxygenation within the cell.

Increase in the amount of energy ATP production in the body, as well.

Like you see it is evident that there are numerous advantages to health that you can enjoy when using this type of therapy as well as other forms of light therapy treatment. It is crucial because we'll benefit many things with these treatments helping our bodies be healed in a more organic way.

There is a possibility of taking many medications to treat this issue, but they will only disguise the cause and mask the signs, and not offer the real comfort we need. If we quit using the medication is when we're likely to feel unwell again. However, with something such as the red light therapy that treats the problem and assists the body to heal itself naturally and feel better quicker, and have better health in a short time. It can also make a huge difference for millions of individuals.

All of these positive physical options that we have mentioned above which are likely to make up the majority of, if not all of the effects users will reap of when using red or near-infrared light therapies to boost their overall health. Consider all the benefits to health that we've discussed previously in this book, along with many others which are still to be discovered. And you will understand how this light can be so efficient, especially in relation to the cell metabolism.

In order to help us understand this: both infrared as well as the red light can reach deep into tissues in the body. This is crucial because it will aid in reducing the levels of nitric acid that is present in our bodies. The healing potential of eliminating the nitric acid, and eliminating it will allow the cells to heal and complete the job they were created to do. In just a couple of sessions using this therapy you will feel relief and transform cells that may have cancer back into normal and happy cells.

Chapter 5: Is Red Light Therapy Actually Safe To Use?

Another question individuals will ask in using the red radiation therapy, is whether or not it's appropriate to use it or not. There's a concern that it could seem odd, or that it is so powerful that there could be a problem. If we take a look at the range of the tasks this therapy can accomplish and accomplish, it's easy to discern the reasons why there may be some concerns regarding the security of this treatment.

One thing to keep in mind is that this isn't an unusual method that's likely to shock you, or cause you to feel like something dangerous that you should be concerned about. The method is made up of lights. Similar to the light that comes from the sun, which can assist boost your mood since it supplies vitamin D, the red therapy using light is likely to provide light in a certain frequency and will provide lots of advantages for your health. The process is as straightforward as this!

Contrary to a number of various surgical or medical treatment options available in today's medical field Red light therapy is safe and has a low risk of negative side consequences. Numerous procedures and drugs have a long range of potential side effects which may be harmful or even fatal in certain situations.

You've seen the commercials where they go over all of the adverse side effects which are associated with the medication which are suggested. They claim to provide you with many positive outcomes, however you must be concerned about negative consequences. Sometimes those side effects are expected to be severe it's not hard to ask yourself if it's worthwhile to try the drug or endure the illness or suffering.

However, with the use of red light therapy, you can expect to experience only a few negative unwanted side effects and a majority of patients experience little or no discomfort whatsoever. If you compare it with different methods available the red light therapy method is considered the most effective treatments, and also among the most safest of all therapies.

Based on the Dr. Michael Hamblin, who is a scientist and professor at Harvard, "In terms of adverse effects, there are only a few adverse effects. There are instances when I've heard of people who used a light to their head. I believe some people had headaches as well as a couple of people who felt overly tired."

They aren't any reason to fret about. There is a possibility of a mild discomfort as you adapt to the detoxification process, etc. when working with the treatment with light. Also, it is possible that you will be required to nap once the therapy has been completed in the event that it causes you to be somewhat sleepy. But you're good! It's based on numerous studies and investigations conducted on a variety of people with no complaints. Most didn't have any of these symptoms at all.

There is a chance that you won't be able to go through the abstracts of the research that has been carried out on red light therapy however, if you look at the studies that is included in this guidebook, and others you'll find there is no evidence of adverse unwanted side effects for the majority of patients that went through these research studies.

One of the main reasons you won't read about many people who have done red light therapy, and suffering negative effects is the fact that the power of the wavelengths of red light is extremely very low. The quantity of exposure will be able to receive by the force of the red light will be such that the body temperature will only be able increase by about 10 percent over the course of your treatment.

It is not a significant increase in temperature and this is great news. This will never result in any type of injuries or burns on the body. As a result, it is possible to utilize this therapy over longer periods of time and never have to fret about injuries to your body as a result of the light.

It is also possible that devices are used for near-infrared as well as red light therapy tend produce a tiny amount of luminescence. Most times it will produce less than 12 Watts of illumination. With this little quantity (a bulb for home light is typically going to have 70 or more watts) You are likely discover that the device has certain incredibly powerful effects that are felt on your body.

Like we said in the previous paragraph as this treatment will have almost no thermal effect on your body, it's an excellent option for those who have an injury you wish to heal. The injuries you suffer from will be more prone to heat, which is why you shouldn't to use therapies which rely upon heating.

In the end, they require some form of treatment with a low amount of temperatures. Higher temperatures are likely to cause irritation of the injured or increase the severity of the injury and make the swelling difficult to control and even worse. The heat source could cause the pain more severe in the procedure. With the use of red light therapy you'll find because there's no need to worry about the heat the treatment is suitable to use in these cases of heat-sensitive injuries.

Finally, if you're worried treatment with red light is not suitable for you as a treatment, it's actually approved by the FDA for several different ailments, and the US Government is adamant about this type of therapy to be suitable for the majority of people.

Although it's recommended to speak with your physician prior to making a make the decision to use the use of red light therapy to meet treatments however, it's generally regarded as healthy. It is able to treat many different medical conditions and will allow patients achieve great effects. Since it's simple to apply, you'll be likely to locate a professional within your region who is knowledgeable about the best way to apply the treatment and who will be able to answer all your queries regarding the therapy as well as assist you through the very first (or hundredth) treatment with red light therapy.

Chapter 6: Creating Space For The Treatment

We now know something about the benefits of red light therapy and the reasons why it's an effective treatment for various diseases, it's now time to study the actions you could follow to maximize the benefits of this treatment.

In this part in this section, we will discuss the five factors you must be aware of when you're preparing to begin your own red light therapy. It includes finding the ideal space to perform the therapy, the correct physique position, the placement of the light source, the frequency of when you need to do your sessions and the duration of the session should run.

A thing to be aware of prior to starting the initial part is that simplicity is the key. This guideline should help make life simpler. This isn't meant to make you feel that there are many details to keep in mind it is important to not think that you must be unsure of yourself all every moment. One rule you should keep in mind and adhere to is to keep things as straightforward as you can. This will make therapeutic sessions more effective as well as enjoyable.

Now that we've got removed the obstacles and we're ready to consider ways to create an ideal space for the treatments. Imagine this in the following in this way: If you had start every session taking the device down three steps then plug it in, and lay on a hard, cold cement floor for 15 minutes or longer, how likely are you to go on with the therapy regardless of whether it actually did produce positive results?

It is possible that the room you select to do the therapy will not be this awful, but it's the best example of what you could do in order to understand the significance of having an appropriate space to serve purposes of the therapy. If you're not able to make the sessions as relaxing and enjoyable as is possible it is likely that it will be difficult to keep going in any amount of duration. The greater the amount of work you'll need to accomplish and the more unpleasant the sessions will be most likely to be, you'll only be able to do treatments for a handful of sessions before giving up in frustration.

That's why it's an excellent idea to make a place within your home or office where you can dedicate yourself to the treatment with light. Actually, it's vital in order to achieve optimal results while you're working on the session. Also, the location you select should be able to ensure that the process itself is easy and enjoyable as it can be.

You will now be able to set it up any way you'd want. There is a possibility that working using a yoga mat blankets, or the spread of a towel across the floor you'll have to lay down or lay down will create a more relaxing environment. A pillow or two is a good idea also. Some people believe it best to make sure you have the option of lying on a bed, or chair to provide some comfort your situation.

Alongside the previous alternatives for ease of use, you can also decide to put a timer into location. Many patients prefer to make use of the timer app on their phones for this purpose and that's acceptable. If you decide to utilize a particular timer solely for the red light therapy, ensure that you place it inside the area of treatment. This will help save time and effort not having to search for it in the future.

A different consideration to consider when choosing an area for treatments is the need for at least one power outlet in the vicinity. The light source must remain connected at every moment during your therapy or if you can recharge between sessions, it will make the process simpler.

Then, you can contemplate what you'd like inside your space for treatment. This is your space that is being set up so that it can allow you to relax and remain focus during your session. Every person will add different items in the session, which is okay. However, you should think about what will make you most relaxed and relaxed. What can help you achieve an optimum focus while you're doing the process of light therapy.

In the same way, with your space to think about, you should also take into consideration what time you'd like to apply the therapy. Most often, you perform it early in the morning or later at night. It is possible to choose the you feel is most suitable for your needs. Both are great timings, but you need choose the one that's will help you get energized in the morning or provide you with some relief at night after an exhausting day.

In particular, some prefer to do therapy early in the morning works best for their needs. Red light therapy will assist you in getting energetic and prepared for the day. It will help you concentration, boost memory and also repair damaged cells. It also helps to rid your body of toxins before you leave for your day. It is dependent on the problem you're dealing with, you might find that the treatment time in the morning will be the most effective for you during the procedure.

There are several benefits of taking a few light treatments during the evening. It is an excellent option to fix any of the damages that were done to your cells throughout the day. Additionally, it can help ease certain tension, headaches and many other problems that are built over the course of your day. This remedy is great for those struggling with stress and other ailments which make it difficult to sleep in the late at night.

The most important thing to remember in this segment is to be in a space that is suitable for therapy and select the timing which is most suitable for our needs. If you're able to achieve it is to set up a space specifically to be used for the therapy. However, make sure you choose an area that will feel comfortable and allow the patient to be relaxed and focused when the red light therapy will be working.

Chapter 7: The Body Position During The Red Light Therapy

In the final chapter, we spent time to look at the most effective spots to arrange the treatments to make you feel calm, comfortable and focused on your treatment. We will now proceed to the next component of this. That concerns the body's posture. How you're will position your body while performing any of your treatment sessions will be crucial. If your body is put in a posture which is uncomfortable and you're not able to completely relax you want, it's likely to last for long before the treatment stops capturing the attention of you and you decide to avoid using the device or reap its advantages for a while.

Keep in mind that we're going to feel more motivated to pursue activities we consider enjoyable and enjoyable. It is the reason we have ensure that we choose a body position that fits our body that feels comfortable but offers us the chance to be relaxed all the way and then be forced to stop. It is good to know that there are three different options you can choose from in order you position your body, while receiving the maximum advantages of treatment with the red light. The three options can be used are lying down, sitting or standing.

The Standing Body Position

There are various products for Red light therapy. They are specifically designed to assist those who are planning to be standing for the entire session. This could include LED lights that can be carried on an upright or in the walls. Also, there are some high-end vertical booths that have a swinging door that allows you to enter and out to help in the treatment.

The idea of getting up to receive treatment might seem like something you should try however, would you really like to be stuck in a single spot for 20-minute period twice a each day, based on the treatment you are receiving? Being in one location for an extended period of time may be uncomfortable due to the burden that is placed on your body. It can be difficult for you to ease into your position and relax as you're able to be so that you can see the effects.

If that is the method you find yourself most comfortable applying during treatment or the one that works best in the room you're in, then you can use it. For the majority of people this isn't going to feel comfortable. You may also find the sitting position for so lengthy time will cause you additional discomfort that you wanted to correct through the use of laser therapy. That's why the majority of patients would choose to work in the two other body positions.

The Sitting Body Position

The other option that is possible to work using is the sitting place. If you're able to relax in a recliner that is comfortable or on a couch it is possible to unwind and relax during the procedure. There are many advantages to working from a recliner as it can feel more relaxed as opposed to standing during the time of the treatment, and you have a variety of options on the best place to sit.

However, there are many those who prefer for a different place of work due to some negatives associated with this type of position. A few of the major disadvantages associated with a sitting position are the listed below:

If you practice the therapy at a desk, you'll need to build up some muscles in order to assist you with contracting and prevent you from slipping fully relaxed.

If you practice the treatment at a desk, it could create a challenge to get your red light a position that will allow you to achieve the maximum amount of healing.

If you are doing the therapy sitting down the therapy can be uncomfortable or uncomfortable. Some people feel a little painful in the course of treatment.

There are numerous advantages to sitting while doing treatment, and it's surely a superior option over standing. It's more comfortable and allows you to unwind and enjoy all the benefits. There are certain disadvantages to this method, and you need to evaluate to determine whether this is the one that is best for you to enjoy all the benefits from the Red Light Therapy.

The Laying Down Body Position

If you're able to accomplish this, then lying down may be the ideal alternative to consider. It is considered to be the most effective method for the treatment of red light therapy. The position of lying down will offer all the ease and comfort you're seeking. It allows you to ease every muscle of your body. It is the only one of three the most secure in case you are unable to sleep during exercise.

Many offices offer the therapy these devices will be suspended in the ceiling, and the patient resting on a massage table beneath the light. That's one method to accomplish this. Locating an over-supportive framework to use as a light hanger may require some creative thinking and effort, but it's an option worth trying.

Chapter 8: The Position Of The Light During Treatment

Another thing to look into while doing some of our therapies is the positioning for the lights. Because you'll find that lying down be the best position for your body as doing your treatments and the majority of concentration we give this will be on where the light is supposed to be when you're lying down. However, before that, let's discuss where you should place the light while you're standing or sitting.

You can first choose to apply light therapy sitting. While standing to receive treatment, the positioning of the light could be or on a standing platform or an illuminated light which is fixed on a wall close to where your. It will help you benefit from the treatment without needing to keep the light in place throughout the treatment. There is however one drawback, which is that you'll need be able to sit up while receiving the advantages.

You have the option of sitting in your chair in a chair while you do the treatment. This can be a great choice, and the ideal location where the light will be placed is placed on a table directly before you or it can be placed in your lap and face your. The position for the light here will hinder your ability to treat any area of the body which is outside of the face and chest, as the distance will be closer for these areas when you select this.

It is also possible to select various lighting options while lying down. When compared to lying or standing positions it is likely that the placement of the light when lying down will make it easier. It is possible to lay on your back in the correct location, and then set the light right next to your body on the floor or on the bed. You can aim towards the region of your body which needs to be treated.

There is the option to suspend the light on a ledge above your head If you think this is the most appropriate option for you. For the majority of people sitting down with the light towards the direction of the region of the body which requires the treatment is likely to be the most effective and most often the simplest spot to position the light.

If you have to work to relieve discomfort in your lower back You can simply place the light behind you to the part that's creating the pain, and let it go. If you are suffering from a painful knee, you can lie on your back with the light on your knee. The same applies regardless of which region of your body you're feeling discomfort or discomfort in, or which kind of treatment you're looking to get. Lay the light red against your area of your body while you rest and take in the light which is reflected when you lie down.

Like we said before, sitting down is likely to be one for body position for your treatment with red light. It will provide the user a variety of benefits but also aiding in light positioning. This is because it has the simple design you require, as we have discussed before and ensures you can relax and unwind when you are trying to make the most enjoyment out of your time.

Chapter 9: The Duration Of The Session

Fourth thing is worth spending the time to consider before we decide to perform an in-person red light treatment is the length of the treatment. It means that the majority of patients must consider the length of time they would like to utilize the red light every time they get started with treatment. The number of times you will use the light during your day as well as the duration of your sessions are going to be contingent on the issue that you're attempting to resolve, as well as the severity of the issue at the time of beginning.

The length of your session will be the amount of time you expose your part of your body to the Red Light. It is possible that you will find yourself trying a few different things and observing what is most effective for you can ensure that you are getting the best duration for each session.

There's some scientific research being conducted to figure out the length of sessions to obtain most effective results. This is based upon the issue you're facing. It's also crucial to be aware that no thing is fixed as a fact. It is possible to take further and then there's the possibility that you'll require less time to get the results. Beginning with the foundation which is discussed in a variety of research is an excellent base to start from however, you are able to alter or reduce your time based on your personal preferences.

If you're worried of being too lengthy for the treatment It is okay to start with shorter or less frequent sessions, and gradually increase to the level you desire. Be aware that the red light therapy method is among the safest treatments and treatments you'll be in a position to use for a wide range of conditions, so there nothing to be concerned about in the amount of time you've chosen to go with the treatment.

The first thing you might consider using this method is to apply the red light treatment on your entire body. If you're comfortable to do this, then sit in a fetal posture wearing no clothing and the light in towards the position right between your stomach and chest. The idea may be awkward however, remember that you're in a room by yourself, and will be an excellent way to get your body for general healing starting.

The purpose of a full body workout is assist you in reaching every cell within your body as possible. In this way, if you practice it the right manner, you'll have the ability to hit the upper arms, chest, stomach and your upper legs efficiently as you can in one go. This is a great option if there is only one light, and you wish to target as many of your body during one session of treatment.

Although you may have purchased the device to treat a specific aspect of your body like painful or injured ankle, it's an excellent idea to spend the time to treat the entire body prior to moving to work on that specific particular body part. This will allow you to experience the power of healing that the smallest device that uses the use of red light therapy can be able to bring the body.

If you opt to deal on your whole body You will be able to feel more relaxed quickly. That's because you're doing as much work on your body's cells as is possible. The first thing you notice is how much better you feel more relaxed, less stressed, and you are able to heal other issues and you can see that things that you would not even have noticed that were causing you pain previously. If you choose to try this type of therapy it is likely the time to focus on this therapy in about 20 minutes the ideal time to begin.

Most people find that using treatments for between 15 and 20 minutes will be sufficient for the effects you desire. However, you might need to play around with it for a few days. Although there's no harm in going a little more time on the treatment plan in the event that you want to, as the only thing it will accomplish is to increase your overall health, without adverse side effects, the majority of users prefer what time of day they like best.

There are two options in this regard: You can choose to start by taking twenty minutes required for treatment or proceed and gradually raise the amount of time until you are at the point that provides your with the greatest advantages. It takes longer, however it lets you be aware of the specific time frame for the treatment using red light which will be most beneficial for the disorder or disease that you're dealing with.

As an example, you could begin with a session of five minutes to see if it works. It is possible that you will find it's not enough to offer all the relief you're looking for and so you extend the duration of your treatments to 10 minutes each day. You can then check how it is working for you. After that, you can add 15 minutes and 20 minutes and on.

There is a chance that you're good with 15 minutes and do not believe there's a lot to be gained by going between 15 to 20 minutes. That means that you are able to choose between two, and pick the one that works most suitable for your needs. When you begin to feel that you are not growing stronger or more effective as you increase the time, it's an indication that the shorter timeframe when you first started to feel like this is likely to be the best one for you.

Furthermore, you might observe that every part of your body might require a distinct period of time. It is possible to feel the relief of an ankle pain within ten minutes, however you may realize that it takes more than 20 or 25 mins in order to ease your anxiety or stress in your daily life. It's normal and taking time to play around can help you discover the timings most suitable for your needs.

Chapter 10: Recurrence Of Sessions By Using Red Light

Fifth thing that we must think about as we prepare to begin our session will be the duration of sessions. It is important to decide the frequency we will need to conduct these sessions. It is important to know if you are doing it a couple of days a week, several times per week or anytime we notice that there is a flare-up and again.

The frequency of sessions will be described as the quantity of treatments you'll have to complete every day or during the each week. In general terms taking into consideration what is effective your best, research has found that a schedule of between 2 and 20 sessions per week are likely to yield results. That means you could have to attend up to three or more sessions per day to get the treatment. Some people prefer to only have a couple of sessions over the course of each week.

You can however select the frequency which will be most suitable for your needs. It's not necessary to be concerned over how frequently you make use of the device however, if you'd like to test this out and do it more frequently than twice or three times per week, that's okay, as it is safe to use red light therapy and won't cause injury with increased usage.

Many people, at the very least getting started with 2 treatments every day is likely be beneficial for their. This will help to repair the cells, and keep them as fit as they can be. As time passes, people could decide to move up or down in the amount of sessions they take depending the way they feel. If you do one before getting up in the morning, to get you going and ready for the day ahead, after which you can do one in the evening to assist you achieve a better restful and restful sleep could be a great option to meet your requirements.

The most frequently addressed here is because the red light capable of reviving the cells in our bodies, is it necessary to be worried about performing the procedure at night or how can it interfere with the rest for the individual? Relax this moment since the answer is not as many patients have reported that completing an exercise session prior to when they sleep can aid them in falling asleep faster and remain asleep during the evening.

The reason is that the red light will reduce the levels of cortisol and adrenaline within the body. This helps people to sleep during the late at night. Furthermore, as the therapy using red light helps us in reducing the level of stress we deal with, it makes it simpler to get sleep.

Before you make any modifications to how you're using for the treatments with red light be sure to test it before you start. It is a good idea to follow all the advice we've discussed in relation to the treatment. Determine the position that the light should be placed at, what direction the light will be placed, how frequently it is recommended to do sessions and how often it is recommended to complete the sessions. The treatment with red light is designed to provide a treatment that is a good fit for you so taking the time to tailor it so that it work for your own personal preference is essential in order to achieve outcomes.

Chapter 11: Common Mistakes People Make When Using Red Light Therapy

If you are considering using treatment with red light and red light therapy, you can enjoy a number of positive benefits you will get: You'll be in a position to improve the strength of your bones as well as aid weight loss, decrease depression and anxiety, understand how to manage anxiety levels, and numerous other. While more research is conducted regarding this treatment will be revealed, nearly everyone is able to benefit from the treatment to restore their health and feel better.

It is crucial to remember that there are some typical mistakes to watch out for while using the red light therapy. It is important to know the best ways to avoid these mistakes so that you can be sure that you maximize the benefits of your treatment, and you don't feel that it isn't working to meet your requirements or specific health issues. The most frequent errors that novices do when they are first beginning to use treatment using red light therapy for health concerns comprise these:

They Don't Do It for Long Enough

The timing of your sessions with light therapy is vitally important. If you do not spend enough time with the light every day, you might not be able to reap the maximum benefit you're hoping to get. This is the reason it's crucial to test a little and determine the length of time the light in red is best depending on your particular condition. For some people, it is possible to complete ten minutes several times throughout the day while others may require closer to 20 minutes or more for similar results. Every person will differ, and this is dependent on how your body reacts radiation.

If you've tried this treatment a couple of times and still don't believe that it's doing anything to your needs, then it's the time to try experimenting a to see if it can help. Test a variety of ways to find the one that is the most effective for you. comfort you require. It could be that when you add just 5 minutes to your workout it's possible to change from feeling nothing to feeling fantastic in just a few minutes time!

They Didn't Do Their Research

Conducting some research on Red light therapy can be a major difference to the way you view your experience are able to have regarding it and what you'll have the ability to utilize the treatment for. It doesn't matter if you're in need of some research facts to decide the effectiveness of this method or not, or would like to learn more about the ways this procedure is likely help the health of your family, you'll be able to find an abundance of research studies as well as more information on the topic.

The most damaging aspect of the lack of scientific research that most people aren't aware of the many advantages they could reap from the therapy. There may be a chance that they have heard of some of the advantages of the use of red light therapy. However, as they've never conducted all the necessary study, they do not realize the possibility to enhance the health of their patients through the treatment. The more you know about red light therapy it becomes clearer how it can be used those who choose to try the therapy.

However, if you've gone through this manual and come across the issue you're looking to fix in the checklist, it doesn't mean the only option is out. Simply, you have to do evidence that demonstrates the advantages of this method that could be for anyone.

They Are Skeptical About the Process

We've been well-trained by big pharmaceutical companies and other people who earn a lot of money in the world of medicine. We are taught that we have to purchase expensive drugs, go through expensive procedures, and risk our health to ensure we will be able to eliminate any illness or disease. This is a big deal for certain companies, however it's not always the right choice for our needs.

We are all aware that the advice we've been given does not serve our good interests. But it makes us skeptical about alternative treatments that are effective, however, they don't fit to what conventional medical practice informs us about. It's a challenge for many patients miss out on a few of the advantages associated from this type of treatment since they do not believe it's a good idea for them or any other person.

There are many wonderful benefits to using treatment with red light. This therapy can help everyone who's will to give the treatment a go. Even if you're not an avid fan of medical treatments or surgery, as well as the standard treatments we are using today, why not give this a shot? There is no risk of adverse side effects and just because the red light therapy is utilized, this doesn't mean you must abandon other things. Why not boost those some? If you're not convinced that it's effective, there's none of the negative side effects, so it might be just the thing you're looking for.

They Don't Learn How to Relax All of the Ways

The most important thing be aware of is that you must remain relaxed while the red light therapy performing its task. It may seem like it's not too much However, you must to be sure your body is not overly stressed and your body and your mind are able to rest for the entire duration of the therapy regardless of whether the treatment lasts 15 minutes, 20 minutes, or 30 minutes or more for effects.

It might be difficult for certain people. It isn't easy to see outcomes from any therapy you choose to try in any therapy you attempt. Stressing all day long can slow down your process and it isn't likely achieve the level of relaxation you'd want.

There are some actions you can to follow that can aid in relaxing. If you're looking to relax, taking some time to perform an exercise in deep breathing prior to getting started, then reading, or perhaps having a bath could assist. It is possible that just only a few minutes of mindfulness can make a huge change. There is the difference when you do the session when stressed and anxious, as well as doing it when you have found the method to let you relax prior to beginning.

Not Choosing the Right Device

Another thing is important to consider when it comes to this treatment is selecting a device which is able to function to provide you with the treatment you require. It is not advisable to choose a gadget that does not use an infrared device or a red one and isn't capable of delivering the results as claimed to do.

It is crucial to conduct an initial study prior to. There are a few high-quality choices of devices available however there are several companies who are attempting to get on board but may not give you the quality product you're looking for. Check the reviews as well as the information that is included with the device to ensure that you will achieve the outcomes you're looking for.

They Don't Put the Light in the Right Spot

This is an straightforward one to solve. It is just a matter of making sure that you've set the lights at a location in which it will be in contact with the issue you are trying to resolve. One of the most challenging situations which arises is when you want to perform the treatment throughout your body however, you're not certain which way to go about getting to the entire body. If you are trying to treat back pain, such as, it's the most effective in the event that you apply it to your back.

Do some research into where to place the light fixtures, as well as knowing how to place it in order to not remain in it all the duration can be helpful. In the case of back pain You may discover lying down on the ground, and getting lighting right in the point that causes pain to your back be the most effective. If you'd like to work in a full-body posture in a fetal position, the one which we discussed in the previous chapter or arranging the lights to be higher than your body and be able to reach all places equally.

Understanding how to use the red light therapy method is essential in order to get positive results along the path. It is a good thing that this method will be secure and reliable and will do great for you once you're ready to treat your body naturally. Pay attention to the typical errors above to ensure that you are as well-prepared to reap all the benefits of treatment with red light.

Chapter 12: Faqs About Red Light Therapy
It's normal to be informed about red light therapy, and you may have questions. A lot of people haven't been aware of this type of treatment and it's quite different from many of the other treatment options and treatments available in the present. However, this doesn't mean that it's more effective however it's crucial to be aware about it. Asking questions is among the most effective ways of doing this. Let's look at some of most frequent questions that people ask regarding using Red light therapy in order for you to see which treatment might be an option that is right for you.

Do you need eye protection for Red Light Therapy Treatments?

The very first thing we're looking at is whether it's necessary to put the eyewear you normally wear while working with the treatment using red light. In the present the patient has not reported suffering from eye issues or eye injuries during the use of laser therapy. Actually, this type of treatment has been proven to improve eyesight and the way they're capable of working.

That means that, as with the rest of the tissues of your body, if you keep your eyes closed and unprotected then it's likely you'll gain the use of this type of treatment within your daily life. The only time it might be advantageous using eye protection is when you are concerned that the intensity of the light is just excessive for you. There aren't negative effects if you choose to simply turn on the lights with no protective measures for your eyes.

What is a Wavelength

As we're discussing the use of light therapy and light and light therapy, it's important to look into what wavelengths are all about, and the reason it's crucial. If we look at electromagnetic radiation like radio waves, light waves that are emitted by this therapy will be able to traverse space which will result in an elongated sine wave. The wavelength that we're trying to find is simply will be the length that the form of the waves will repeat. In this case, for instance, the red light used for this treatment is less in terms of wavelength than near infrared. On the other hand, far infrared is a wavelength that is much longer.

What Kind of Bulbs Are the Best for the Treatments?

There are many alternatives to consider in the course of your treatment, and finding out which one is the ideal for your requirements is crucial to be sure that you are seeing improvements of your treatment. In the beginning the incandescent light and halogen lamps will produce around 35 percent of the strength they provide in the same range used as a treatment with light.

The lights you choose will be ideal that you can work with. They are different. They release a small amount of UV light, however they are not expected to emit any ultraviolet light. they'll emit any infrared, red or near-infrared light. This is the reason we are typically going to suffer adverse effects after exposing our bodies to light sources, when compared with the red light therapy. These lights have been identified as major contributors to some of the most harmful health conditions and diseases that individuals across all of the United States are fighting.

Why Are Near-Infrared and Red Lights Better Than Far Infrared Lights?

Near-infrared and red radiations which's wavelength will be anywhere between

500nm and 1500nm. They will be taken up by an enzyme located in the mitochondria of cells. This enzyme was discussed previously, which is known as "cytochrome c oxidase". It will lead to a larger quantity of energy produced by this cell compared to cells that aren't struck by light.

The need for energy within cells as it is what makes a cell is healthy. If you can have enough cells to generate the energy they need in a timely manner that is, it will be easier to stay healthy. However, this isn't something that we can expect to be able see using the technology of far-infrared. This type of light will not absorb or be utilized by enzymes. this causes it to function in a different way.

In looking at infrared far-infrared lighting it is evident that their wavelength is much longer than other lights. It can range from 1500nm up to 10,000nm. This is because the infrared light unlikely to strike cells, providing the cells with energy. It is instead going increase the metabolic rate of the body, by causing a the body a slight increase in temperature within the body.

Thyroid hormones are accountable in regulating body's temperature. If the thyroid hormone isn't working as it should increasing the body's temperature using other techniques could help improve metabolic rate. One reason we might need to consider this is because reducing the temperature overall of our body, even only by one degree could have an impact on the activity of enzymatic enzymes. A lower level of activity indicates the body's metabolic energy production will be affected.

The meaning is that when the temperature of your body falls below what is considered ideal, the use of an infrared sauna helping to improve the efficiency of the enzymes, ensuring that the metabolism can be expected to improve throughout the body.

Is It Normal to Feel Some Tingling During the Therapy?

A few people have complained of feeling sensations of tingling performing this treatment. Based on the doctor Dr. Michael Hamblin, this sensation is normal. It is visible on the skin following treatments at times, and it's really just a dissociation photochemically of the nitric oxide when it begins to break away from the cytochrome C oxidase enzyme inside the cell. The treatment is achieving exactly the thing it said it would, and you'll start experiencing the effects in no time.

How Does Pulsed Red Light Therapy Work?

Another option to be thinking about while using laser therapy that is red, would be the concept using pulsed laser therapy. The process will almost exactly identical, however instead of having the light remain steady on the region of the body you want to treat, you're likely to see the light flash between frequent intervals throughout the treatment.

The principle behind the pulsed red light therapy basically a switching on and off the red light with an exact frequency to create flashes. This treatment will alter the cell similarly to continuous wave therapy has been discussed in this book, and it accomplishes this by increasing the ATP production inside mitochondria within cells.

However, some are looking to determine if pulsed light therapy is either more than conventional treatment. If you compare these therapies, you'll find inconsistent research. Certain studies will show that the light that pulsates is the most efficient, however, there are some reports who claim that the continuous light is the most effective.

One of the studies which was recently conducted to examine the relationship between the effects of pulsed therapy versus regular therapy was conducted by Dr. Michael Hamblin. Dr. Hamblin was able to compose an exhaustive review of these treatments and also took time to examine the effect of different frequencies in order to determine which one would perform best and whether or not.

The main thing that was revealed in this study is that both methods are effective. What is important is to use the red light. It doesn't matter how it's pulsed, or not. The patient will reap advantages in all cases. If you decide to utilize the pulsed therapy, be sure your pulse is steady and slow, not too much. If you let the light move too quickly you are likely create confusion for the cells, and result in losing any benefits.

The majority of patients who choose to opt for pulsed therapy will find the frequency between 10HZ and 100HZ is the ideal way for starting.

The decision to choose pulsed lighting will depend on your preferences. It is up to you to decide if you feel more at ease using the constant light as opposed to the pulsed light and which is giving you the best advantages. Be aware of your body's needs and trying a few experiments along your way is the ideal decision, irrespective of the method you choose to use the therapy with red light.

It's normal to have many concerns when using treatment with red light, no which method you decide to choose or the problem you wish to treat. Be sure to go through this article and address all questions you might must ask to ensure you are fully aware of all the ways this treatment can help you.

Chapter 13: Strategies For Accelerating Your Healing Through The Use Of Light Therapy

We now know something about red light therapy as well as everything can be done using it, it's an ideal time to dig deeper into some of the options you're being able to accomplish to make this treatment truly become a reality and perform many things for your health.

Although the therapy with red light can be extremely effective by itself however, there are some actions you could do to further enhance the results. The actions you take are usually easy, yet they will propel your progress and make the results more rapid and better. A few of the methods you could follow to reap the maximum benefits of treatment with the red light include:

Do Two Sessions a Day

It is possible to only do only one treatment per time if you want however, many patients find that they're getting the best benefit from their treatment in the event that they can take two or three sessions over the course of the course of the day. It is important to try different things and find out what works most effectively for you.

If you opt to perform the treatment with light at least once per day You are doing your best to repair the cells, and also keeping the Nitric Acid out of your body. You will be amazed by the change it makes. It will be like you feel you are more energetic inside of you once it's time to begin your day as well as beneficial to wind your body into a relaxed state after a hard day's doing work and taking care of the additional obligations throughout the rest of the day.

Naturally, you will are able to determine that one treatment can do what you require or it difficult to schedule the sessions multiple times, you can stick to the quantity of sessions that meet your requirements. However, many people who utilize this treatment and get great results will really enjoy doing the bright red light at a minimum of a handful of times throughout the every day.

Get Plenty of Sleep

Another thing is important to consider this is taking your time to sleeping regularly. If you're lacking sleeping, you're not providing your body with the time to replenish itself, or clear out the harmful toxins that afflict the body. Although you may be using the therapy of red light, when you're not getting sufficient sleeping regularly and your body won't get rid of the toxins it has accumulated out, which means you're likely to be feeling less well.

In reality, sleeping enough every night isn't easy for a large number of individuals. It is important to learn how to manage your health and get off the phone and decreasing the stress levels in your life are vital in order to fall asleep during the night. Some of the methods that you can achieve to achieve a quick sleep and sleep through the evening include:

Stay at work If you are a frequent visitor to the work you do at home and work from home, it's going be a challenge to learn to sleep at the right time. A lifestyle like this usually results in stress and may not be able turn your attention when you are ready to sleep.

Switch off all electronics before going to sleeping: If it is possible you can turn off your electronics at least an hour prior to going to sleep. This can help to cleanse your brain of the light that is emitted through the cell phone, computer as well as other electronic devices, so it can rest. Think about writing, reading, or resuming your routine for bed in this period instead.

Create a list of items you have to complete in the coming day. It's hard to fall asleep when you're surrounded by millions of thoughts and items to keep in your head. When you go to bed, create your list of things that you'd like to accomplish, so you do not need to think about remembering these things later.

Make sure you are active throughout the day. If you're sitting in front of a computer all the time, or don't do anything, it could be difficult to maintain the level of activity you are putting in. To avoid letting this take place, look for ways to become more active to ensure that your brain is prepared for bed. If that's doing more exercise and exercising more, or establishing a fitness schedule, you must discover the way of doing it that is the most beneficial for you.

Create a bedtime routine A routine can be an excellent way to signal your brain it's time to shut down and get ready for bed. Starting this process a bit prior to bedtime will have a major impact too. It is possible to make it either as long or as short and as simple or as complex as you prefer. Keep the same routine for each day.

Shut off the lights The darkest night is generally the most relaxing. It assists in signalling to your brain that it's the time to fall asleep. Locate any light which are present in the area that might keep you awake during the late at night, and work out the best way to shut them down or remove these lights.

There is no TV in the bedroom It is a common practice of people who prefer to lay down with a TV in their bedroom. They believe this will help people fall asleep during the time of night. Even though you may have the ability to fall bed with the brightness of the TV on, your rest will not be as deep. Shut it off or move it off the wall to see the effects it could bring to your.

Take a moment to listen to a quiet or soft music, if you need to There are people who find or the sounds out of their windows are high or they aren't comfortable in silence. If this happens for you, don't make it the reason to head to the TV. Instead, you can turn on gentle classical music or music that is accompanied by the natural world, and let it help to soothe your mind to sleep.

Sleeping enough is essential for you to reap the full positive effects of treatment with red light. It's not easy to achieve this, but placing yourself first, as well as knowing when you can not accept other commitments and desires can simplify the process.

Eat Lots of Healthy Foods

For your cells to be healthy If you wish to reap the maximum benefits of the treatment with red light it is essential to be more conscious of the food that you consume. Do not undergo the therapy with red light and afterwards indulge in chocolates and frozen ice cream for the duration. Instead, filling your body with nutritious foods that are healthful and provide the body with the nutrients that it requires to stay healthy as well as to make necessary repair, will be vital.

The question is about how to consume your food in a healthy method.

It is not necessary to stick to a strict eating plan or adhere to a plan which is difficult to stick with. If you're looking to lose some weight, while you are doing this treatment, then that's acceptable, however, by eating food that is healthy for your health, and produced using real ingredients instead of processed ones, you will get better results too.

In order to ensure you're eating food which will keep you full and ensure that you're getting the nutritional benefits you require, consider food items in their natural state. A diet that is full of fresh fruits and vegetables, as well as lean sources of protein and meat and using healthy oils for cooking, dairy products without added sugars, as well as whole carbs from grains can help. Find out how to eat portions that are appropriate, and learn to tell your body's signals to know if it's hungry or not. Then, you'll start seeing positive changes in the health of your body as well.

Learn How to Get Rid of the Junk

It's acceptable to indulge in a little bit of junk food at times whenever you want something sweet but we all consume lots of sugary treats and unhealthy food items that aren't needed. There are a ton of sugars, carbohydrates baked items, juices and sodas as well as many other things. This is very bad for our overall health.

If you're looking to decrease your problems in your body's cells, and other ailments, you must aid the treatment with red light to work by removing some of the unwanted substances. You should limit yourself to some of them occasionally, instead of creating it into a routine in the diet you follow. It can be difficult and may require you undergo some sort of a cleanse to help this happen. However, if you're capable of sticking with it program, you'll observe significant improvements in your overall health.

Drink Lots of Water

It is important to be sure you're taking all the harmful contaminants out of your system through this process, and maintaining your hydration and ensuring that all organs and components of your body function properly. We often become too distracted by our lives, or drinking pop, coffee or other beverages, but we don't make sure that we will have the ability to provide our body the proper hydration requires drinking water.

The goal should be to drink the minimum amount of 8 to 10 glasses of water each day. If you're still thirsty following that, go for a run, or experiencing an extremely hot, try to consume more. This will aid you in getting maximum benefit from treatment as you can as well as a more water throughout the day is enough to make you be more comfortable.

Try to Avoid Stress (As Much as Possible)

If you've read this article and you squirmed and shook your head, you're not the only one. There is constantly more than enough anxiety and stress for us to handle in our current world. Trying to figure out ways to reduce stress, or even reduce it to the extent feasible, could seem something that is impossible to accomplish. The more you can reduce and reduce stress within your body, then the healthier your body will become in general.

There are many options perform to lessen the anxiety you feel throughout your day. A few of the most effective suggestions comprise:

Learn to decline: It's commonplace for people to get into the pattern of saying yes every time somebody asks them. Be happy if are already occupied and aren't able to assist. Know when you are able to do more or when you simply cannot take it on.

Take a few minutes to meditate: even an hour or two working on the gentle therapy will help ease your mind. Eventually, you'll feel anxiety levels melt out until you're not able to feel the stress.

Enjoy a relaxing bath. It can help relax your mind and may help spur cells to increase power and speedier recovery.

Have a time with friends It's not difficult, when you consider everything we have to do throughout the day to become too distracted to take a step back and focus on the relationships require. slow down and find ways to create greater connections, have more time and get more connected to your friends as well as your family.

Fitness: A few minutes of training can be a great help in detoxifying the body. It will also help you achieve even greater results.

Find something you love to do It will be apparent that just a little bit of time in the morning to pursue something you like can lower the amount of anxiety you're likely to experience.

Stress is not an ideal thing to do for the overall health of your body, so it's ideal if have strategies to lessen the effects of stress. By following the above steps, and figuring out what works most effectively for you, will guarantee that stress levels remain to the low level.

There's already a myriad of benefits when you do some treatment with light. However, when you include these examples and ideas that we discussed in this section, you'll realize that it's easy to recognize healing and good overall health you'd like and all it takes is some Red light therapy during the course of your day.

Chapter 14: Tips To Get The Most Out Of Your Red Light Therapy

We have spent quite a bit of time getting to know about the benefits of red light therapy, and the many amazing benefits it can help you improve your overall health. We have spent time studying the numerous advantages to health that are associated with this treatment, as well as the various ways you can utilize it to make sure the red light is in the correct area of your body in order to complete the job it was intended to do, and many more.

With some of the information removed from the equation we can examine a few suggestions that you should apply to ensure that you get the maximum benefits from the therapy options available. You are likely to get some amazing results applying the light to your body and leaving it in the dark for a few minutes every time, there are handful of suggestions and tips you could follow to allow you to get the most benefit out of every single session you take. The tips can be helpful with treatment with red light comprise:

Be sure the lighting device is used provides all the spectrum of white light. It is also insuring that it's equipped to block all ultraviolet light. It's ideal if the light box can block out all of the radiations since they're regarded as extremely harmful to your body.

Set the box up so that the box is level with your eyes or even higher. Its position and the size of the light box relationship to your eyes will affect the way you see. It is important to make this light box simulate what you would see if you're outdoors in the sunlight.

The box should be placed to ensure that it is only a few feet away in front of your eyes. It's best to place the box about two feet away off the eye at the time you use it. However, if you already know the lighting in your box has a little less power than you would like, you'll need the light to be moved closer. This method will perform best when the box you have is an 10000 Lux box. The distance should be adjusted based on the dimensions of your box this level.

Maintain the light box in a way that it's at an angle rather than straight across. There is a chance that keeping the light box at either about 10 or 2 degrees is the most effective way for you to reap the advantages. It's not recommended to put the light on your eye or in the exact spot that you're trying to solve. It is recommended to place it in a way that the light is 45 degrees to from either direction from the middle of your eye.

Choose a lamp which is around 10,000 Lux. It is not advisable to use a standard lamp as you'll not see the light red that you get from this. 10,000 Lux makes the lamp strong enough that you will enjoy these benefits and at the same time, not have worry about whether it is excessively strong or insufficient enough to work with.

Keep up with your use of the container: It's recommended to utilize the box on a consistent schedule to achieve the most effective outcomes. If you are only using it when you're thinking about it or somebody else reminds you of the issue, this is not the best thing to do. The result is that you'll be missing all the amazing things that could occur when you regularly use the red light therapy and you're unlikely to be as awed by your results. getting.

If you're on certain medicines at the moment discuss with your doctor regarding using the therapy of light. It's not likely to create too big issue, however certain medications might not behave in the manner you'd like them to after a red light has been placed on their. This could mean that the medications make your skin susceptible to light, and this may alter your appearance of the skin, which appears like a rash, or sunburn. Talk to your doctor and determine whether this could be a concern to you, or otherwise.

Select a timing that is the most effective for you. You need to select the time slots that work most efficiently for your needs. If you're deciding the time between evening and morning, and both or decide between five or twenty minutes, you must choose a period that works well with your daily schedule in terms of time, duration and the thing you're most at ease with.

Choose a great physique position. You must be able to choose a suitable place to perform the therapy with light. In general it is advised to do the gentle therapy when lying down. If you decide that either sitting up or standing is the ideal choice for you, proceed with this choice. It is important to remember that you must choose the most comfortable position for you. most relaxed, and can enable you to fully relax. If you're unable to be relaxed and at ease with the therapy, it's impossible to enjoy the benefits once you have started with your Red light therapy.

Check the state of your health or mood following the red therapy with light to determine whether it's working. Just a couple of moments of the therapy are sufficient to increase your mood. It could be noticeable immediately after completing in the session. Sometimes, it could take a few days after therapy, when you begin to feel an improvement. It will be easier to feel better more relaxed, less stressed and more energy in general.

Use this method in conjunction with alternatives that we've discussed in this book for the most effective result you can get. Incorporating other treatments such as those that were discussed above will allow you to truly benefit from the red light therapy.

Utilizing the red light therapy will prove be among the greatest things you'll achieve to improve your health overall, whether your goal is to reduce weight, relieve the pain in your body, aid in cell repair, boost your memory and so many more. Understanding how this therapy functions as well as implementing some of these tips for treatment is likely have a significant impact to the way you experience.

Contrary to some medications you might have used previously or the ones your doctor as well as others have discussed taking you off at some point in the near future, you'll have the ability to utilize laser therapy, and will not need to be worried about adverse side consequences. It will give you the advantages of a healthy lifestyle and less pain, in addition to many other advantages and all using a way that's healthy for the person you are. Consider how good you will feel by simply applying Red light therapy consistently by following the guidelines we have discussed in this article!

Chapter 15: What Is Red Light Therapy?

Beauty is an important part of the women's personality. Therefore, a large number of women worry about the negative effects of ageing. Many women are trying anti-aging creams and other products in hopes of regenerating the appearance of their skin, and making it appear younger. However, they generally fail.

A recent study has revealed that a particular type treatment can regenerate the skin's tissues and bring back its youthful look. This revolutionary concept described"the Rejuve Anti-Aging System, and it utilizes the groundbreaking Red Light Therapy to combat age-related effects, wrinkles, dry skin and dry patches on your skin.

The skin lotions and ointments which advertise anti-aging qualities usually do not result in an improvement on the skin of the person using them as they focus on areas that are not visible to the skin. It is because the product's objective is to cleanse the pores and help make your skin appear more radiant by creating the appearance of a uniform complexion. There is a chance of turning back the time on the skin's appearance are not that great in the absence of tissues that are completely renewed.

Researchers have found that the red light reaches into your skin. It causes a beneficial change in the skin due to the increase in production of collagen. Collagen is the primary protein your body needs to heal and repair damaged or torn tissues. One of the main concerns on people's minds right now is whether this method of treatment is completely safe.

There is one minor difference, the method of this special kind of treatment is similar with tanning. This particular type of treatment can be found in a room or bed. It's done similar manner to how the tanning process is carried out, however the distinction is that this kind of treatment involves glowing red tubes, which produce none of the ultraviolet radiation or light sources, meaning that people seeking to take better the best care of their skin don't need to be worried over UV radiation. It's quite easy to get this kind of therapy and is a great way to turn around and look younger.

Chapter 16: The Benefits Of Red Light Therapy.

Have you considered the value of using treatment with red light can be to both beautify and for medical procedures? The technology was developed to offer a viable alternative to those who are averse to using medications to treat medical conditions.

It is possible that you are interested in the origins of the red light therapy. The therapy has advanced and is used for rejuvenating the skin, and regenerating cells in order to eliminate wrinkles, facial lines, and acne from the 1950s onwards. The therapy is also used in order to delay the aging process. The treatment with red light provides vitality to the cells of your skin and activates them, while decreasing the size of pores at the top of the skin. Every day, the procedure lasts about 15 to 20 minutes.

The red light therapy may be employed for important reasons for medical use, including the reduction of pain and inflammation within the body. It can be a great alternative to the use of drugs to those suffering from fractured muscles, broken bones and tendonitis. It can also help with strains, injuries, arthritis, and Fibromyalgia. It is a great option for those who do not like taking medicines due to medical reasons.

There are many options for purchasing an red light therapy device however, make sure it's approved from the FDA (Food and Drug Administration). In the event that you don't, and are wasting moments with this device, it's not going to improve your health. The therapy device is available in many styles. It is hand-held, which is one that is the most economical. However, after about 15 minutes of holding it and sat down, you'll be tired. If you'd like to work on an area that is larger it is possible to use huge lighting fixtures for overhead lamps.

In the case of treatment with red light for pain relief, it is different from aesthetics with respect to the duration. To get the most effective alleviation of pain, plan to make time for 30-45 minutes. In addition, you could supplement this treatment by doing some gentle stretching exercises. Massages can help to relax joints and stiff muscles in the course of therapy. Additionally, the treatment with red light isn't fast fix. Instead, it is suggested to use it for at minimum 10 times. It is recommended that you get one of your own since you'll spend less money in the salon or in a medical facility.

Chapter 17: Red Light Therapy For Skin Quality And Happiness.

The stimulation of collagen can occur by a number of different methods to keep your skin looking great. Vitamins E, A, and C, in addition to the various acid treatments, and IPL are great for stimulating collagen. A majority of these therapies depend on inflammation in order to improve cell turnover in the skin and consequently increase the volume of skin however there's another fantastic solution under the "Stimulating Collagen label that will cause no harm to your skin at all.

Even though the treatment with light has been in use since the beginning of time yet it's considered the latest technological advancements in skincare. It is because of the possibility that the red light treatment may help in reducing signs of aging, such as wrinkles, dry skin and so on. Similar to the way plants use photosynthesis. Red light triggers the natural chemical reactions inside cells that may trigger cell turnover as well as the formation of elastin and collagen fibres Similar to the way plants use chlorophyll to convert sunlight into building blocks for cells. The creation of ATP within mitochondria of the skin can be triggered by red light. In turn, mitochondria produce energy that stimulates the production of cells. This release of energy enhances the growth of healthy cells that can then be replaced by cells damaged. Contrary to other treatments using light, like IPL or Laser This procedure doesn't use heating to damage the dermal layer instead of giving energy to cells. It is important to know that this treatment does not emit UV radiation, which makes absolutely safe, with no reported adverse consequences.

In the past the use of light therapy for years has been used in medical environments for wound healing and with the price of the equipment is decreasing Spas and beauty salons are starting to offer this service. The spectrum of light therapy for anti-aging is 615nm and 640nm. It creates RED light. The brain's receptors are activated through light that emits particular frequencies. Different frequencies trigger different reactions. Red light has been found to enhance the growth of collagen as well as elastin inside the skin as well being able to reduce signs of ageing and sun damage. Tests conducted by clinical researchers in collaboration together with University of Pavia revealed a 20.2 percent decrease in the volume of wrinkles as well as the result was a 24.7 percent improvement in moisture levels on the skin as well as an 15.1 percent improvement in the smoothness of skin. The visible spectrum of light can be used to deliver light to the epidermal layer to aid in the process. If the light energy gets delivered to the skin is activated, the body triggers an activation reaction called photomodulation. The light energy is absorbed into the cells, and is then dispersed to stimulate the body's cellular collagen production processes, leading to rejuvenation of the skin and improved general health. If you undergo these treatments every each week for about 4-6 weeks, you'll see a change in your skin's tone and appearance at the close of your treatment. Recognizing that the red light therapy requires time to achieve its effectiveness. Be aware that you're not just reversing time, but you are also slowing down aging.

RED lasers were initially created to treat skin and face, however red light is now offered in collagen beds, which could be utilized to treat the all body. This is a thrilling advancement because typically we devote lots of our dollars and time on facial skincare, but doing nothing for other parts of our bodies. When you get older and especially around fifty You'll see your skin begins to lose weight all over the body. The collagen beds can slow down the process of aging. They have been called"the "next big thing after Botox." The benefits are numerous such as the alleviation of headaches, and improved circulation of the blood, due to the fact that RED laser relaxes blood vessels and allows increased circulation. It is also utilized for treating depression as well as the seasonal affective disorders (SAD). Utilizing light therapy may also aid in treating strains and soft tissue injuries. Each day new benefits are discovered, including reduction of the negative effects of dysfunctional sexuality, even though this claim may not be backed by an established scientific basis at present.

Personal experience suggests that it is possible to feel very relaxed following the procedure, and it seems to boost the mood. This is the perfect treatment for me. Amazing appearance and a sense of happiness together. It's amazing how little people know about the benefits that are so amazing of RED laser therapy.

What Are the Real Benefits of Red Light Therapy? Does Red Light Therapy Work?

What Are the Benefits of Red Light Therapy for Your Skin and Body?

A Little Backstory

Therapy with light has existed in numerous forms throughout duration. Indeed, Hippocrates, an ancient Greek doctor, was well-known to educate patients about the benefits of sunlight and advised that they expose themselves for exposure to light in order to treat various illnesses. Recently it was scientists from National Aeronautics and Space Administration (NAS) found the use of infrared and red LEDs (light emitting diodes) treated lesions at significantly faster rate when conducting study of plant growth within space. The power of light has been exploited and extensively studied since that findings, and has shown a wealth of medicinal and beneficial benefits.

Nowadays, treatments using red light is available in clinics for dermatology and chiropractor's offices, doctors' offices, spas salons, clinics and even in homes. While this procedure becomes increasingly well-known, some might be skeptical and ask how effective it is.

It's Yes!

Chapter 18: What Is Light Therapy And How Does It Work?.

The wavelengths created by LEDs (also known as light emitting diodes) (LEDs) measure in nanometers. The more intense the wavelength and the more deeply the light can penetrate the body more the number of nanometers. Particular nanometer wavelengths are being studied and have been proven to penetrate tissue, skin joints, bones, joints in which light is absorbed by the level of cells. The healing wavelengths have over 24 beneficial effects when they are absorbed. These include:

* Improving blood flow

* Enhancing the production of collagen and elastin.

* Restoring cellular vitality (ATP)

Encouragement of the healing and repair procedures

* Increase the quantity of endorphins released

* The nerves that transmit pain are blockage.

Skin and body are the result of these changes that take place in the tissues and cells.

Here are a few benefits of skin care:

The reduction of wrinkles and wrinkles

* Crow's feet reduced

Age scars and spots aren't as apparent.

* A silkier finish

* Pores that are less

• Skin is more tight and more firm

• A younger appearance

* Increased collagen synthesis and elastin

• Redness lessening

*Relief from rosacea

* Blemishes heal more quickly

* The inflammation is lessened

Here are a few advantages to health

* Pain relief

* Injuries heal more quickly.

Edema and inflammation are lessened.

* Extension of the mobility

* Increased circulation of blood

* Nerves that send signals to the brain are blockage.

* The production of endorphins is increased.

Which wavelengths will work the most beneficial for skin rejuvenation? And what wavelengths work the most beneficial for relieving pain?

Yellow LEDs that have an average wavelength of 590 nanometers, red LEDs that have the wavelength of 625 to 660 nanometers and infrared light sources that have a wavelength of 830nanometers or more can go through all the layers of skin to heal and repair the damage that has occurred previously.

For alleviating pain the red LEDs having an 660 nanometer wavelength and infrared light sources with 880 nanometers of wavelength are able to penetrate as much as 2 inches deep into skin joints, tissues, and bone, alleviating discomfort and speeding the healing process.

Treatment with Red Light is a highly effective method of improving skin appearance as well as alleviating chronic and acute discomfort. It's an entirely non-medicated efficient, secure, and effective treatment option for many illnesses.

Which home automation systems are proven to be effective in real life?

Best for Rejuvenation of the Skin:

The DPL Therapy System is a dual-panel hands-free device with red LEDs 680 nanometers, and infrared leds with 880 nanometers.

Quasar MD is a powerful device that uses five millimeter LEDs that have four wavelengths of 640 nanometers and 660 nm. It also has 880 num, and 940nm.

Baby Quasar Plus It is a handheld gadget that has three-millimeter LEDs with the 640-nm range, 660-nm 880 nm, 940 nm. The unit is less bulky than the Quasar MD.

ReVive light Therapy Beauty Kit - This unique handheld device has two heads. One of which emits red light at 625 nm, and an infrared one at 830 num. Another head is equipped with blue LEDs of 415 nanometers which are designed to destroy the acne-causing bacteria P. acnes.

Another hand-free panel includes an alternative to the Caribbean Sun skin rejuvenation Light made of the red LEDs of 660 nm and green LEDs at 590 Nm.

The most efficient methods of pain management include:

DPL Therapy System Two-panel hands-free therapy system does not just rejuvenate the skin, it also includes LEDs to reduce discomfort and speed the healing process. The panels are removable and securing to different areas on the body.

ReVive Light Therapy for Pain ReliefIt is a handheld device that has red LEDs which have a wavelength of 660 nanometers and infrared light sources that measure 880 nanometers long in wavelength.

DPL Flex is a flexible belt with a few pieces that fit into pockets. It's simpler to put to more areas of your body due to it being elastic. Red LEDs that have the wavelength of 660nm as well as infrared LEDs that have the wavelength of 880 nanometers are utilized in every panel.

Chapter 19: Treatment And Tools For Light Therapy To Help Delay The Signs Of Aging.

There is no doubt the fact that gorgeous skin is attractive. In a time when the majority of girls and women have beautiful skin, it is a fact.

For men, there are anti-aging products and lotions which promise to eliminate facial imperfections, including those unsightly wrinkles that indicate the age of your face, while other are seeking out costly consultations with a doctor as well as treatment options that could cost as much as they can be uncomfortable.

Cosmetic procedures to smooth out wrinkles, lines and wrinkles are seen as excessive ways to remove cosmetic imperfections. Technology today, contrary to what you might think allows you to achieve a more youthful radiant, more glowing complexion free of dark spots or uneven tones. The perfect and glowing skin is yours when you are aware of the right equipment and cosmetics to apply to suit your specific skin type and preferences, saving you suffering in the form of thousands of dollars as well as the time to recover.

Nowadays, cosmetic treatments using light and laser therapy has become an increasingly used process.

today. It's not cheap obviously due to the complexity and technological requirements.

They require the manufacturing of the machines. The efficiency of these machines can be proven.

nevertheless.

The use of red light therapy, as an instance, can speed healing time for scars as well as wounds that are on the skin.

When compared with any other medication more cells are able to work effectively on the skin, if blood flow is increased which results in better the growth of tissues. The red light is absorbed quickly into the dermis, which is why it's gentler and more efficient over visible infrared lights.

NASA has tested the technology before and discovered that it is beneficial, not just for healing wounds however, it can also be beneficial in treating various skin conditions like the eczema outbreak, acne, the scarring process, and rosacea. Light therapy can aid in improving conditions of the skin by stimulating the growth of cells and also removing the harmful toxins on the skin. They are hard to get rid of using soap and water.

The best part is that this breakthrough technology is being utilized in many products available on the market.

BrightTherapy provides a range of products that help both women and men to improve their appearance and rid themselves of the common ailments.

It is not just that the BT Trident SR11A Light Therapy System include only one head of treatment.

Three distinct kinds and each one will treat a specific skin problem. Red Light Therapy is a kind of light therapy that makes use of red light

As an example, a massage to the head can help reduce wrinkles and lines. Also, it improves appearance, texture and tone of your skin. It makes your appearance younger and more radiant.

Its Blue Light Therapy head is designed to combat the causes of acne and other problems by eliminating bacteria from the skin. This provides an immediate remedy for oily skin, while tightening the pores.

As the heads can be swapped so you benefit from the device since you receive Green Light Therapy to help reduce sun damage, discoloration hyperpigmentation, or discolouration on your face. The BT is, without any no doubt, the top.

Its Trident SR11A- Light Therapy System makes a fantastic accessory to every bathroom cabinet. It is also possible to try an attempt to the Light Pad LED Light Therapy System a shot. The Bright Pad LED Light Therapy System is a light source.

offers the benefits having the anti-aging equipment you want. are available in Red and Blue

It may help remove signs of aging, such as the appearance of dark spots, pigmentation and wrinkles.

wrinkles. In addition, it aids with the treatment of acne as well as the prevention of hair loss.

Latest advances in the field of light therapy.

Chapter 20: Does Red Light Therapy Really Work?

Elastin and collagen, two of the components of your skin's structure break down and become degraded when you get older, which causes the skin to exhibit signs of ageing. Exposure to sunlight and pollution, gravity, cigarettes, harsh soaps along with free radicals and poor nutrition all accelerate the degrading of collagen and the elastin. Everyday, you as well as your skin are bombarded with harmful substances. There is however an easy, painless method to prevent the look of ageing without causing any negative side consequences.

What exactly is red-light therapy and how can it be used?

The treatment, which is also called photo rejuvenation is a method that uses visible blue light wavelengths of 630 - 660 nanometers as well as infrared wavelengths that are 880nm or greater to get deep inside the skin's layers, boosting cell energy and encouraging collagen and elastin production. Due to their concentration of blood and water the skin's layers absorb light very quickly. Photo rejuvenation is now one of the most secure quick, fastest and economical methods to achieve remarkable anti-aging effects on the skin.

Does red light therapy work?

LEDs (light emitting diodes) with Infrared and red wavelengths provide incredible therapeutic benefits on living tissues as demonstrated by research carried out in the last forty years. LEDs have been proven through studies that they cause some 24 beneficial effects on a cellular level. They help support healthy skin cells that appear younger.

The appearance of wrinkles, fine lines and large pores. skin, and crow's foot are all known to be effectively treated with photorejuvenation. LEDs create major changes to the skin's surface at a sub-dense layer, healing collagen, cells and elastin, with a gentle and safe method.

Light therapy using red has been around for a long time (LED light therapy)

NASA invented LED lighting technology to aid in research on the growth of plants It was then found to be effective to speed up healing space. The doctors began to experiment with LEDs at hospitals for treating injuries, and discovered that the red and infrared light sources boost the energy levels inside cells as well as boost mitochondrial function (the cell's powerhouse.)

Skin cells when subjected to light the cells grow between 150 and 200 percent faster, speeding the process of healing and repair that allow the skin and body heal and repair damage from the past as well as current.

Benefits of the Red light therapy

It reduces the appearance of wrinkles and lines.

The appearance of Crow's feet

Increases the speed at that imperfections can be repaired.

Improved skin tone.

The production of collagen and elastin is stimulated.

Skin damaged due to sun damage is fixed.

Enhances the natural hydration and elasticity of the skin

Increases blood circulation to the skin.

Reduces roughness on the skin.

Pore size decreases.

Texture is softened.

Skin degeneration is slowed.

Redness and flushing throughout, and capillaries that are dilated are lessened.

There's no risk or discomfort, but only beautiful and more gorgeous skin.

Treatment with red light therapy is not just effective in fighting against ageing, but is also safe for the skin like that lasers may. It is suitable for all types of skin Non-invasive, treatment that is not ablative (skin-damaging) without time-consuming downtime, painless, and an easy procedure. The light wavelengths are gentle on the tissue, skin and cells, helping to promote healthier skin, tissue and cells, without causing harm. One of the very few methods that are non-invasive and can actually combat the signs of aging is the treatment using LED light.

The pain is alleviated with treatments using LED light.

The reduction of discomfort, muscles and joint pains, sprains back pain, and sprains have been shown by LEDs to be effective. The wavelengths of the red and infrared light can penetrate deeply into the body, easing the pain and repairing injured tissue. The wavelength of infrared light, 880nm, penetrates to depths of 30-40 millimeters. This makes it extremely effective in treating issues in joints, bones as well as deep muscles. The red light of 660nm penetrates the skin at a depth between 8 and 10mm. This makes it helpful for the treatment of injuries, cuts or scars as well as infections located closer to the skin.

Cognitive performance can be improved through treatment with light.

It was just discovered to improve cognitive function after brain injuries sustained from trauma in a landmark research. The daily light therapy treatment applied on the scalp and forehead at home has been proven to enhance cognitive performance in a dramatic way which includes memory, inhibition and the ability to hold the focus and concentration of one's attention.

Red light therapy help treat many skin issues as well, but it can help to ease pain and aids in cognition enhancement. This is a fantastic technology, which is still being studied and discovered to offer amazing health benefits for the body, the skin, and the brain.

CHAPETR SEVEN

Red Light Therapy For Anti-Aging.

The treatment known as red light, also known as photo-rejuvenation, is an LED light therapy that is used to fight aging. In order to promote healthier and younger complexion, this treatment makes use of Light Emitting Diodes that are specifically targeted towards the skin. The treatment with red light is completely organic and causes the body to react by increasing your skin's appearance by nourishing it from within.

NASA has studied and designed the product for skin care and first utilized to study the reactions of plants against LEDs. This procedure proved that it increased cell growth, and eventually proved beneficial to human cells. Even though human and plant cells do not have the same characteristics however, light of the appropriate frequency has been proven to boost skin health in a natural way.

Red is the colour of healing. It's employed to treat various of ailments. This includes the management of pain (back strain, pain and tennis elbow). ...). It is better when it is combined with the infrared light source, since the infrared light penetrates further. When it comes to skincare, your skin absorbs the light which increases the production of elastin and collagen. Both of these proteins are crucial for softness and firmness of your skin.

The production of collagen and elastin decreases when we get older The small veins that transport vital nutrients and blood from the bloodstream onto the skin's surface are much smaller. Light therapy with red wavelengths rejuvenates cells, and makes veins able to transport greater amounts of blood and nutrients for your skin.

It has the effect of cumulative. In the end, the more you utilize it and more, your skin gets more supple and soft. Face treatments usually last from 15 to 30 minutes. However, you could focus your attention at specific parts of your face like crow's feet and the corners of the lips neck and more. Lines and wrinkles become filled with collagen once more You'll feel relieved to see your skin regain its natural glow and tone.

Another form of treatment using LED lights also known as blue light therapy is utilized for treating acne. Hyperpigmentation can be treated using green light therapy.

Its beauty is that it does not require procedures, and that you won't require as many creams and lotions as many people believe. Equipment for red light therapy that was previously available only through dermatologists, clinics for skin as well as spas, are accessible for purchase by the public at large which allows you to have treatments from the privacy of your house. Prices for these equipment is variable ($100 to $400) however it's worthwhile when you think about the savings you'll make for other products to treat your skin and how much cheaper you'll be than having to go to the office of a dermatologist.

Chapter 21: How Red Light Therapy Can Make You Look Younger?

The Red light treatment can create an element of magic to the skin, triggering over 24 positive biological reactions. Yellow, red, and infrared light sources are beneficial in promoting a healthy, youthful, and healthier appearance. Every LED color comes with an individual penetration level which is the case with infrared and red LEDs piercing deeper into tissues and skin more than yellow LEDs.

Sunburns, rosacea and eczema may all be addressed with the help of light bulbs that are yellow. The LEDs can help reduce the appearance of edema and redness while improving the appearance of skin. Light therapy using yellow has been proven in numerous studies to reduce wrinkles and wrinkles. This Caribbean Sun Light combines red and yellow LEDs in order to help promote the appearance of youth and a healthy appearance.

Collagen production, healing of cells and circulation are stimulated with the red light. Skin cells are able to absorb light in a way that is efficient due to the high level of water and blood in your tissues, which results in a strong rejuvenation of your skin as well as cellular renewal. The use of red light therapy can help diminish wrinkles and lines and age spots as well as acne scarring and encourages a better skin tone in addition to other benefits.

Infrared LEDs penetrate further into tissue and skin more than yellow and red LEDs. They combat the signs of aging through speeding the healing process, replacing dermal and epidermal cells and kicking repair process into high gear. DPL Therapy System DPL Therapy System combines red and infrared light sources in one, hands-free device to help promote skin that is younger looking that is less wrinkled and wrinkle-free.

The production of collagen and elastin decreases when we get older, cell turnover decreases and UV-induced damage is more apparent. In the meantime, free radicals and gravity destroy your skin creating a look of age and dead. The use of red light therapy is proven to assist natural processes function more efficiently and appear as they were younger, thus slowing down the signs of ageing. Collagen as well as elastin comprise the two vital proteins found in skin, which give it bounce, suppleness and aid in preventing wrinkles. The production of both these essential proteins using the treatment of red light, which results in more firm skin, with less wrinkles.

These are just a few positive aspects of using red light therapy

* Reducing the look of wrinkles and lines.

* Reduces pore size

* Enhances the texture and tone of the skin

* Brown spots are diminished.

* Aids in healing sun damaged skin

Reduces scarring

* Reducing the appearance Redness

* Increases the production of collagen.

While aging is inevitable but you can make steps to help your skin appear more youthful and vibrant using methods like the red light treatment. The treatment of red light is used to help many women and men appear younger, without harsh procedures for more than 40 years. It is a procedure that can last for a for a long time and will enhance the appearance of your skin.

Chapter 22: 15 Benefits Of Red Light Therapy For Your Skin.

The use of red light therapy has become ever more sought-after by professionals and non-specialists trying it. However, what is the real magic behind this simple technology and what does it mean to improve your skin?

While light is long known to be calming, NASA only recently revealed the fact that LEDs with infrared or red wavelengths are not only therapeutic however they also significantly reduce the pain and speed the recovery process. The findings prompted a flood of study into the potential advantages of treatment with red light.

LEDs (light emitting diodes) at precise wavelengths have been found to induce positive changes in the cellular levels as per scientific studies. The wavelengths of LEDs can be easily absorbed by the skin and tissues because of their high concentration of water and blood inside the body. In this way, they enhance cellular power, increase collagen and elastin production and improve circulation. They also speed up recovery, initiate repairs, increase oxygen into the area being treated as well as many other.

How do you determine the cause of all these reactions? Your skin is likely to appear more youthful as it repairs past injuries, and improve the appearance of your complexion from the inside out when it's treated using the red, yellow or infrared LEDs.

Your skin will look younger, more radiant and healthier as the changes occur as time passes. Benefits are numerous and it appears that the list will grow as more and more tests are carried out to demonstrate the potential of LEDs.

Skin Benefits of Red Light Therapy

1. Reducing wrinkles and wrinkles

2. The size of the pores is decreased.

3. The skin tone evens out

4. Age spots diminish

5. The skin is firmed and tightened.

6. It reduces the appearance of redness.

7. Relieves the appearance of rosacea-related symptoms.

8. This reduces the amount of time for the blemishes' to be treated.

9. The redness, pain and inflammation is reduced.

10. The skin's texture is smoothed.

11. The production of collagen and elastin is stimulated.

12. The swelling is lessened.

13. Makes glowing skin.

14. Scarring fades

15. The skin appears more youthful.

The treatment with red light is a secure, efficient method to enhance your skin's appearance without any risk of pain or discomfort. The treatment is generally offered at spas, salons and doctors' offices, and at your homes with devices for personal use.

If you are looking for a top-quality and efficient home device look the LED wavelengths that are within the established spectrum (for instance, yellow around 590 nanometers and red at 625-625 nanometers, or infrared wavelengths at 880 nanometers or beyond). The wavelengths penetrate the tissue and skin in different ways. The greater the depth of penetration and the deeper the penetration, the more powerful the nanometer band.

There is a huge number of houses available which is rising as more and more people are conscious of the many advantages that the Red light therapy can bring. How do you determine who are able to trust?

In the first place, this is an investment in the health of your skin appearance, self-esteem, and beauty. If you think a product is going to be cheap but it's likely to be a disappointment compared to the expectations you have set. The one that has high-end LEDs that are in exact nanometer range will cost additional. There are some devices available that have established track records, come from reliable companies, with real-world proof of its effectiveness.

Additionally, you can pick between a handheld model as well as a hands-free panel. What you must think about is the type of system you're likely to choose. It is necessary to shut your eyes when using the hands-free panels to give your face a complete treatment. Your eyes can remain open during treatment sessions using the handheld device, however you'll need to shift the machine to various areas on your face.

Since the LEDs are more to each other and their wavelengths don't disperse as much since the unit's head sits right on the skin. studies suggest that handheld devices can be more powerful over panel systems.

This is a time of excitement as the red light therapy can allow the improvement of your skin swiftly and effortlessly with powerful rejuvenating LEDs. It's a straightforward technology which is great for skin, and the home-based systems make it affordable and easily accessible.

Chapter 23: How To Give Yourself A Spa-Quality Red Light Peptide Facial At Home.

Did you hear a lot concerning LED Lighting Facials recently? Given their safeness and efficiency, they're fast becoming a sought-after beauty treatment. What exactly are they and how do use them for your benefit?

Red light treatments for facials are in fashion!

The red light therapy facial is highly sought-after because they're a safer alternative to more invasive and possibly harmful treatments. This is a relaxing method to effectively cleanse, rejuvenate and rejuvenate your skin, while stimulating collagen and elastin formation and repair UV damages, and encouraging the appearance of a gorgeous appearance. But what exactly is the red light treatment for face?

In order to increase the speed and efficiency of effects of anti-aging from the LED wavelengths, the light therapy facials include a treatment with light that combines yellow, red or infrared LEDs, and an peptide serum based on light.

Particular wavelengths, like red between 625 and 660 nanometers as well as infrared between 850 and 880 nanometers have been found to penetrate into the tissues and skin, and when coupled with a peptide serum results in the peptides getting pushed further into the deeper layers of skin. There they can help to repair and heal the skin, as well as stimulate over 24 positive cell response.

Can you do these at the comfort of your own home?

They are not just offered at the top skin clinics doctors' offices, clinics, and spas. The beauty of this method is that it can be completed at the comfort and privacy in your house. Benefits of this powerful technology are extremely easy to take advantage of with devices made for use at home. For instance, the DPL Therapy System, reVive Anti-Aging Light Therapy, Baby Quasar Plus, Quasar MD, and the Caribbean Sun Skin Rejuvenation Light are all FDA-approved, professional-grade products that offer a simple easy, quick, and efficient solution to provide your skin with an expert-quality facial at the comfort of your own home. These are the most effective devices that are available to use at home, and FDA approval assures you that they're both reliable and safe.

Just relax as your skin is absorbed by the reparative effects of light and then responds with a gorgeous glowing. The application of a peptide serum that is light driven prior to LED treatments increases the benefits, and also cuts short the amount of time for results dramatically. The peptides have been proven to provide significant benefits for skin that are a benefit to the skin. When used together with light treatments and light therapy, they're pushed deep into the skin which can offer additional help.

Are they true? do the job?

Certain wavelengths of LEDs have experimentally proven to create cells with energy, boost the rate of metabolism, boost the production of collagen and elastin, and start a chain of healing processes within the cells and tissues. The activity of fibroblasts is enhanced through red light within the range of 625 to 660nm and infrared lights in the 850-880nm region that stimulates them to produce greater collagen as well as elastin. If you add peptides into your mix, the collagen production and skin firmness, luminosity as well as skin smoothness as well as a host of additional benefits explode and produce greater results.

Why do they get so much acclaim?

Faces with red light therapy are gaining a amount of attention due to their simplicity and that they provide outcomes without irritation, redness or pain. There is also no time off. When a reliable LED light therapy treatment is coupled with the Peptide Serum that is Light Driven Peptide Serum the effects are far more dramatic and the procedure is quicker, leading to more healthy skin.

Treatments with red light therapy can be done within a brief duration (9-25 minutes) which makes them perfect for those who are on the move or working a full agenda. This is a fantastic method to make your skin appear younger and more attractive with no pain or discomfort caused by other treatments. create.

What Should You Be on the Lookout For?

If you are looking for a reliable product, be sure to check regarding the wavelength nanometer range, FDA approval, and whether the serum specifically designed for use using a light-treatment device. It is possible to restore a healthy, youthful appearance without surgery, easily, and painlessly without any interruptions once you've got a gadget in your possession.

Chapter 24: The Top 3 Acne Red Light Therapy Devices.

Acne is a skin problem that is a problem for 85 percent of those aged between 12 and 24 including adult acne sufferers to the pile. There are a myriad of treatment options for acne that it's difficult to locate one that suits everyone's skin. It seems that light treatment is the most universal solution and now you can purchase an acne light therapy device to use at home. A majority of patients get benefit from treatment with light which is why this single investment is drawing many people to. Here are the top sought-after skin light therapy devices that are portable in this piece.

Let's start by defining one thing: the light therapy to treat acne is actually a blue LED light. The devices emitting this shade of blue light can be effective secure, painless, and safe. The red light also is used as as the best light therapy method to treat skin issues as it can address a variety of problems (acne and aging skin, dry ...).

Blue Ageless Beauty Marvel Mini It costs $225, and is highly appreciated by the people who use it. The device was so popular that many online beauty shops promptly ended up selling out. Marvel Mini devices are also accessible to treat aging (red laser therapy) as well as hyperpigmentation (green light therapy).

Baby Quasar - Baby Blue. Baby Blue was created to complement the red light therapy device Baby Quasar Original. This is an extremely powerful product that customers say aids in treating mild to moderate acne. Baby Blue, at $349 Baby Blue, at $349 it's a little expensive as the red and blue light therapies is recommended for treating acne, you may require an additional device. (The Original Baby Quasar costs $449.)

Tanda Skin Care System is a top-quality skin care product. It's probably the most effective option. The price is $395 this isn't exactly pocket cash. The Tanda light therapy apparatus includes two different modules that can be used that is blue-colored light therapy, as well as the other one to treat the red light therapy. Tanda Clear (blue light) is able to eliminate acne-causing bacteria, whereas Tanda Regenerate (red light) helps to heal the skin, and minimizes the appearance of scars in addition to being anti-aging.

The process for using an instrument for treatment with light is simple and consistent. All you need do is switch it on, and then shine the light onto your skin for about 3 to four minutes. This isn't UV or laser light, which means the light won't harm the skin. Of course 100% natural since it does not require usage of chemicals or medications to perform its function. The bacteria are eliminated by the blue light since it's taken up by it. It is evident after just a couple of days usage, and your skin will clear over, and your complexion is flawless when you combine it with the red light therapy.

Chapter 25: Types/Sources Of Red-Light Therapy

Red light therapy is performed in a variety of methods. It is explained in the following paragraphs.

Spas and facilities for medical use:

The majority of medical spas across America as well as Europe provide services like massages and red light therapy, among others. These facilities do not provide tanning beds-style with red light equipment and the bed is not a source of dangerous ultraviolet radiation. They employ licensed health practitioners who supervise the use of red light therapy.

Light bed in red.

Domestic installation:

The benefits of the Red light are attainable when it is installed in the place of home for fast and simple access. A hand-held device is also utilized. The device is placed on the affected part of your body. Others kits include red lighting lamps, light bulbs and other devices that are designed specifically for use on the face that are identical to a mask for face. To ensure a long-lasting result It is recommended to do the exercise early in the morning, and later at night in order to boost mitochondrial function and the production of collagen.

Face mask for hand light therapy

Computers and phones:

The advancement in technology has enabled to use Red light therapy using phones as well as computers. Apple phones have a feature which turns the entire display red by emitting different wavelengths of light. These create an effect on the human body's cells to aid in healing as well as pain relief.

Chapter 26: Benefits Of Red-Light Therapy
Solution for acne and eczema:

The use of red light therapy may help ease conditions of the skin like wrinkles, acne, eczema scars, etc. Red light therapy can reduce the impact and can further aggravate breakouts of acne and eczema on the skin. It is recommended to limit the usage of the red light on your face to keep dry, flaky skin.

Treatment to treat Stiff and painful shoulder

The use of red light therapy in conjunction with exercises can help reduce discomfort and stiffness at the shoulder area.

Enhances sleep

A different interesting aspect about Red light therapy is the fact that it helps improve the quality of sleep and mood. Red light therapy is a regular part of therapy can increase the production of dopamine in the brain.

Recover wounds

A red light therapy can trigger cells to fulfill their job, making it highly effective in healing wounds and damaged skin. Fibroblasts are a kind of human cell body that produces both collagen as well as extracellular matrix that essential for healing of wounds.

It helps improve blood circulation

The red light therapy can help increase blood vessel size to allow for easier flow of blood throughout the body. A lack of circulation of blood throughout the body may cause irreparable damage to cells and tissues.

Enhances the production of collagen Fibers:

If Red light is absorbed by several layers of the skin at a particular wavelength, it causes the creation of collagen and creation of capillaries. Collagen is an amino acid that helps in elasticity of skin. If collagen production is in a good place it will leave the skin unaffected by wrinkles and signs of aging.

Aid in reducing fat levels the body.

Regular exercise and a healthy diet and Red light therapy could lead to the loss of weight. The red light therapy causes an increasing the speed of mitochondria that generate energy, and then circulate it across the body. This is when the body expels more waste out of the body.

www.ingramcontent.com/pod-product-compliance
Lightning Source LLC
Chambersburg PA
CBHW060223030426
42335CB00014B/1318